Speech-Language Pathology

Services in the Schools

Speech-Language Pathology

Services in the Schools

JOYCE S. TAYLOR, Ph.D.

Chairperson
Department of Speech Pathology and Audiology
Southern Illinois University at Edwardsville
Edwardsville, Illinois

GRUNE & STRATTON
A Subsidiary of Harcourt Brace Jovanovich, Publishers
New York   London   Toronto   Sydney   San Francisco

Library of Congress Cataloging in Publication Data

Taylor, Joyce S.
  Speech-language pathology.

  Bibliography
  Includes index.
    1. Handicapped children—Education—Language arts.
  2. Language arts—Remedial teaching.   3. Communicative
  disorders in children.   4. Speech therapy for children.
  I. Title.   [DNLM: 1. Language disorders—Therapy.
  2. Speech disorders—Therapy.   3. Education, Special—
  United States.   4. Speech therapy.   5. Language therapy.
  WM 475 T243s]
  LC4028.T39   371.91′4   81-4221
  ISBN 0-8089-1385-9   AACR2

Grune & Stratton, Inc.
111 Fifth Avenue
New York, New York 10003

Distributed in the United Kingdom by
Academic Press Inc. (London) Ltd.
24/28 Oval Road, London NW 1

Library of Congress Catalog Number 81-4221
International Standard Book Number 0-8089-1385-9

Printed in the United States of America

In memory of Jamie

Contents

Acknowledgments

My appreciation to a number of individuals must be expressed. First, I thank those instructors who responded to my request for course outlines. I am also indebted to Dixie Engelman, Barbara Kent, Marie Taylor, Lynn Taylor, and Mary Wissel, who were kind enough to read the manuscript and concerned enough to offer constructive criticisms. Dixie Engelman, who assumed many of my administrative duties during the preparation of this text, deserves additional thanks. Sharon Bensa must also be recognized for her meticulous typing of this manuscript. I am also grateful to the editorial staff of Grune & Stratton, who made my first attempt at writing a book a pleasure. Finally, my appreciation goes to the students, at both the elementary and college levels, who continue to endure the phases of my professional growth.

Preface

I first became aware of speech and language specialists when I was in fifth grade. Two boys in my class stuttered. Each week, when the loudspeaker announced that "the speech teacher" was in the building, the two boys left the classroom. As I recall, no one in the class reacted to the announcement or to the fact that the boys stuttered. We also had a mentally retarded girl in class but she was never seen by the "speech teacher," nor was a boy who could not talk above a whisper because he had "screamed too much." If any of the other students had communicative disorders, I was unaware of them.

My next recollection of "speech teachers" comes from my junior year in high school. During a career-night presentation, I was impressed by a man who was in private practice as a speech correctionist. Two years later, I entered a university program in speech therapy. The lack of significant interest in the field at that time was reflected in class size; some of my classes contained as few as two students. Following completion of the baccalaureate degree, I began work as a public school speech therapist.* In that role, I experienced problems that we still encounter today: inadequate physical facilities, restricted budgets, lack of parental involvement, and insufficient training in the various pathologies. I recognized the latter problem after only one semester in the schools and returned to school on a part-time basis to pursue a master's degree. Five years, seven student teachers, and one M.S. degree later, I left the public schools for a final encounter with higher education.

The experiences that I had had during my years in the public schools served me well as a Ph.D. candidate; for example, I was able to apply the supervisory skills I had gained in the schools to supervision of student clinicians in a variety of settings. In fact, one observation made while I worked in the public schools served as the hypothesis for my doctoral dissertation. Delinquent tendencies ap-

---

*By now the reader will have noted three different titles used to identify the speech-language specialist; there are many others. The problem of this variation is addressed in Chapter 1.

peared to be the rule rather than the exception in many of the children I had served while in certain schools; my research question was whether the incidence of communicative disorders among delinquent youths was higher than that found among individuals not so labeled. Using an incarcerated population, my observations were confirmed. I was unable to find a direct relationship between specific kinds of delinquent behavior and various communicative problems, but the incidence of 84 percent was significant.

Following completion of the Ph.D., I accepted a university teaching position. My responsibilities included supervising student teachers and teaching the course in public school methods and materials. As I visited students working under the supervision of state-certified speech clinicians, I was struck by the variation in professional competence. Most clinicians were applying the newest techniques and appeared to have a grasp of current thinking. Some clinicians, however, appeared to persist in using ineffective procedures despite a lack of results and without any clear understanding of why the procedures did not work. Further, techniques of case finding and case selection sometimes seemed inappropriate. The only way to counteract these perceived deficiencies, it appeared, was to provide preservice training to students that would ensure their competence as public school speech and language clinicians.

During the years that I have taught the course in public school methods, I have searched for a text that would be both current and usable. In my view, such a text need not provide extensive information on the various communicative disorders; that material is well covered in a variety of books. Nor should a text claim that there is only one way of managing such logistic details as program scheduling. Instead, it should present sufficient information to make school speech-language pathologists aware of various options and to enable them to make informed and justifiable decisions. Federal regulations concerning the management of handicapped individuals must also be considered in such a text.

Finding no book that met my criteria, I surveyed other instructors of courses in public school methods and materials to see if they also felt a need for a better text. In January 1980, I sent a request for course outlines to the directors of 200 training programs in speech-language pathology; both programs accredited by the American Speech-Language-Hearing Association (ASHA) and randomly selected, nonaccredited programs were included. Of the 95 responses received, 55 indicated that such a course was offered by their departments. Almost without exception, instructors indicated that an appropriate text was not available, and many stated that they did not use a text at all. Surprisingly, the outlines provided were fairly consistent with regard to substantive content, although they did show variation in the sequence of presentation of materials.

After a preliminary discussion with the editorial staff of Grune & Stratton about writing a text for the preservice preparation of public school speech-language pathologists, I requested input from other training programs. I have attempted to include information that the majority of instructors deem important.

The order in which materials are presented is one I have found workable, but I have divided the chapters in such a way as to allow for variations.

Chapter 1 reviews the history of the profession briefly and discusses the evolution of the training and professional designation of speech-language pathologists. The impact of federal legislation on the communicatively disordered child and implications of this legislation for speech-language pathologists are considered in Chapter 2. Chapters 3 through 7 take a chronological approach to the school speech-language pathologist's responsibilities in the areas of direct intervention. Case finding, case selection and management alternatives, and program scheduling are discussed in Chapters 3, 4, and 5, respectively. Chapter 6 describes the *individualized education program* required by PL 94-142 and the procedures involved in the development of such programs. Actual delivery of services is discussed in Chapter 7. Although the various roles of the speech-language pathologist in the school are considered throughout the text, Chapter 8 deals specifically with counseling and supervision. The utilization of supportive personnel is discussed in the final chapter (Chapter 9).

Joyce S. Taylor, Ph.D.

Speech-Language Pathology

Services in the Schools

1
Speech-Language Pathology: History and Evolution

Possibly the oldest written reference to speech disorders is a word, included in a papyrus of the Middle Egyptian Dynasty, approximately 2000 B.C. The word has been translated as meaning "to speak haltingly" or "to walk haltingly with the tongue, as one who is sad."

Demosthenes' speech disorder is well known. He has usually been identified as a stutterer, but some feel that his problem could be more clearly described as articulatory. Whether his difficulty was one of fluency or articulation, in the absence of trained personnel, Demosthenes reportedly took it upon himself to treat his own communicative disorder. The success of his "pebbles under the tongue" or "shouting above the roar of the sea" techniques is unclear, but it would appear that Demosthenes presented the first known example of self-treatment for a communicative disorder.

THE ORIGINS OF THE PROFESSION

Stories of individuals with communicative disorders as well as the development of treatment techniques from Pre-Renaissance to the mid-1960s are recounted by Margaret Eldridge in *A History of the Treatment of Speech Disorders* (Eldridge, 1968). Although the absolute accuracy of some of the

---

*From *A History of the Treatment of Speech Disorders* by M. Eldridge. Edinburgh: Churchill Livingstone, 1968, p. 4. Reprinted by permission.

material may be questioned, Eldridge has offered a chronological picture of the development of the field now recognized as speech-language pathology. She has given the reader some idea of the techniques and procedures employed over the years by those treating communicatively disordered individuals. To provide a perspective from which to view the evolution of the speech, language, and hearing professions, highlights from her book are presented here.

Pre-Renaissance to 1900

In earliest times, concern appeared to be afforded individuals with fluency disorders and impaired hearing; lesser consideration was given to other communicative disorders. With regard to stuttering, Aristotle and others felt that inaccurate movement of the tongue was to blame. Apparently this assertion was accepted by others for years. Aristotle also contemplated the fate of the deaf. Although he was accurate in associating congenital deafness with the inability to acquire language, he expressed pessimism concerning their habilitation. Accordingly, the "deaf and dumb" were excluded from society for thousands of years. Throughout the pre-Renaissance period, the tongue was considered the main organ of speech, and its abnormalities, according to the thinking of the time, could cause stuttering. No significant contributions to the current understanding of communicative disorders were made during this era.

Greater scientific strides were noted from the sixteenth through the eighteenth centuries. Human anatomy was studied, and research and experimentation flourished. Among the contributors of the sixteenth century was Ambroise Paré, a French barber-surgeon; Paré was especially recognized as a designer of prosthetic devices, including an obturator. Paré was apparently a caring man whose interest in his patients did not diminish after the preparation and fitting of the prosthesis; in fact, Eldridge (1968) describes Paré as possibly the "first rehabilitation practitioner in history."

Work with the deaf was prominent during the seventeenth century; both manual and oral forms of communication were employed, and divisiveness between those advocating one technique over the other developed. Stuttering continued to be viewed as a disorder resulting from faulty lingual control. Some attention was given to speech following glossectomy and to vocal disorders accompanying hearing impairment.

During the eighteenth century, the first public school for deaf children opened in Germany, and oral communication was emphasized. Little attention was afforded deviant vocal quality, among either deaf speakers or individuals with cleft palates. Although surgical procedures for managing the latter condition were employed, there are no indications that speech therapy was undertaken following surgical intervention. The causes of stuttering remained obscure although Moses Mendelssohn suggested stuttering was due to a "collision between many ideas, flowing simultaneously from the brain" (quoted in Eldridge, 1968, p. 36). This theory differed from any that had been previously proposed. Continued study of persons who had had glossectomies was apparent during this period.

Investigation of etiological factors and treatment possibilities for stuttering advanced in the nineteenth century. Theories relating stuttering to neural debility and to psychic disturbances were among those advanced. Treatment options ranged from breathing exercises to surgical intervention. Even though surgery was dangerous and painful, a great many people underwent surgery to seek relief from stuttering. A variety of theories were proposed during this period, and it is not altogether surprising that therapy based on those theories did not differ significantly from some techniques employed today.

With regard to other communicative disorders, advances in the areas of cleft palate and deafness were made during the nineteenth century. More sophisticated surgical management of palatal clefts was introduced, and obturators were improved. Although the controversy over oral versus manual communication for the deaf continued, instructional procedures for both became more precise. Surgical removal of the larynx was first accomplished during the nineteenth century; rehabilitation in the form of esophageal speech was apparently not attempted. Research in the area of acquired language disorders also advanced during this period, and physicians and researchers such as Brain, Jackson, Broca, Wernicke, and Head came into prominence. The etiology and nature of acquired language disorders were the concerns of these investigators; they gave little attention to rehabilitation.

During the period from the Renaissance to 1900, investigation into communicative disorders was carried out primarily by physicians. Further, educators and elocutionists assumed responsibility for most habilitative-rehabilitative procedures undertaken. Europeans extensively studied speech, language, and hearing impairments; Americans were less involved. Near the end of the nineteenth century, Dr. John Wyllie published *Disorders of Speech*. This book was apparently the precursor of the many volumes on communicative disorders available today.

1900 to Present: The Initiation of Speech-Language Programs in the Schools

During the early years of the twentieth century, classroom teachers were involved in the treatment of communicatively disordered children. Frequently, the assistance given to children involved placement in a special classroom. In Germany, for example, stutterers were placed together in a special room for both general education and speech therapy. Similar accommodations were provided for children with articulatory disorders, cleft palates, and delayed or disordered language development. It is not clear how teachers assigned to these classrooms were trained. Outside of the school setting, elocutionists and voice teachers appeared to have the major responsibility for working with individuals with speech, language, and hearing problems. In the United States, individuals with communicative disorders apparently had to seek assistance from private speech schools; Eldridge (1968) described such schools as being "essentially commercial, as well as secretive in character" (p. 58).

Chicago was among the first cities in the United States to offer services for communicatively disordered children in the elementary schools (Moore & Kester, 1953). In 1910, the decision to provide speech services to children in that city's schools was apparently based on complaints from parents of "stammering" children. These parents asserted that the schools were doing little to help their children; they felt that aggressive action should be taken. At that time, 1287 children were reported to be "stammerers." Later assessment determined that not all of the students had fluency problems; some presented other types of communicative disorders. Before assuming positions in the schools, 10 promising graduates of the Chicago Teacher's College were given "additional" training. Their pay was $65.00 per month. Meanwhile, in New York City, a survey was conducted to determine whether a need existed for speech training in city schools; although the survey was made in 1911, a program was not established there until 1916. In 1916, a survey of the communicative abilities of school children in Madison, Wisconsin was conducted; an incidence figure of 5 percent with inferior abilities was derived (Black, 1966). On the basis of these findings, Smiley Blanton, Director of the Speech Clinic of the University of Wisconsin, suggested that a need existed for special teachers who were conversant with anatomy, physiology, and psychoanalysis. Presumably, these teachers were to work with the speech-defective population. In 1923, the State of Wisconsin acknowledged the need for itinerant teachers; within several years, programs were initiated in large cities on both coasts.

After 1924, programs for the communicatively impaired developed and expanded rapidly. Irwin (1949) provides an example of such program development in Ohio: services were initiated in that state in 1912, but before 1945 there were only seven speech therapists in the state. Following passage of a state special education law in 1945, an increasing need for such professionals was recognized; in 1947, 36 therapists were employed, and this number increased to 46 by 1948. It is assumed that program growth in other states paralleled that in Ohio.

Influencing the expansion of programs in Ohio and in other states was legislation governing the provision of services to the speech, language, and hearing-impaired school child. By 1959, 39 states had some law pertaining to the provision of services in schools (Black, 1966). Today, school districts have little choice; federal law mandates that children with communicative handicaps must receive appropriate assistance from a certified professional.

QUALIFICATIONS OF PUBLIC SCHOOL PERSONNEL

As reported earlier, the first public school speech therapists in the United States were teachers who had received "special training"; Blanton suggested such special training should include background in anatomy and physiology and an understanding of psychoanalysis. Many states establishing requirements for public school speech specialists agreed with Blanton that these professionals should be knowledgeable in the area of the anatomy and physiology of the speech and hearing mechanisms, but an understanding of the principles of psychoanalysis was not considered important. Other areas of preparation did not receive such consensus.

Haines (1965) analyzed state certification requirements in terms of academic and clinical specifications; he reported inconsistencies in many areas. With regard to the degree required for certification, for example, 41 of the 45 states offering a certificate required a baccalaureate degree; only 4 required work beyond the bachelors level. The required number of academic hours in speech, hearing, and related areas ranged from 12 to 51. A 200-clock-hour clinical practicum requirement was specified by 18 states, and student teaching was required in 35 states.

Another attempt to evaluate the consistency of state certification requirements was made in 1979 (Taylor, 1980). A request was sent to all state departments of education for certification and procedural information. Responses were received from 47 states; because 2 states required licensure and one appeared to have no certificate, the requirements of only 44 states were analyzed.

Comparing 1979 standards with 1965 standards, an upgrading of requirements is apparent. In 1965, only 4 states required work beyond the bachelor's level; the 1979 survey revealed that 14 states required the master's degree exclusively. An additional 12 states awarded certification at both the bachelor's and master's level, and 13 states continued to award certification after completion of only the baccalaureate degree. With regard to the number of academic hours in speech, language, and hearing, in 1979, the minimum number of 12 hours had not changed: one state continued to require only 12 semester hours in the major areas. The majority of states specifying semester hour requirements, however, had increased the requirement. The range in 1979 was from 12 to 78 semester hours in speech, language, and hearing; the average number of hours required was 34.63. Clearly, an upgrading of requirements is reflected. In 1965, 18 states required 200 clock hours of clinical practicum; one state required 220 hours and one state, 100 hours. Other states were not specific in their requirements. The 1979 survey revealed that two states required only 150 clock hours, eight required 200, and 14 required more than 200 clock hours. Clock hour minima were not reported by the other states. In 1965, Haines reported that 35 states required student teaching for certification; only 26 states in the 1979 survey indicated that student teaching was required for certification and, of these, just 11 specified the clock hours. This discrepancy in reported student teaching requirements could reflect differing materials furnished to the two investigators. It is doubtful that student teaching experience is required with less frequency today than it was in 1965.

In analyzing the current information on the certification of public school speech-language pathologists, it is apparent that requirements are not consistent. Members of the American Speech-Language-Hearing Association (ASHA) have devoted many hours to the study of minimum requirements for the preparation of competent speech-language pathologists and audiologists. When comparing the requirements of different state certificates to ASHA requirements for the Certificate of Clinical Competence in Speech Pathology (CCC-SP), little conformity is seen. ASHA is specific in its requirements in the basic communication processes area; few state certificates even designate the amount of coursework to be completed in that area. Similarly, a breakdown of coursework in the major area into speech and language disorders is not apparent in most certificate requirements. ASHA requires that all applicants for the CCC-SP have coursework in the area of audiology; only 13 of the certificates analyzed in the 1979 survey have requirements that equal or exceed ASHA specifications. Finally, in the area of clinical practicum, ASHA requires a minimum amount of experience with children and adults who display all types of communicative disorders. Although some states suggest that applicants should have experience with persons displaying a variety of problems, and some even designate clock hour requirements in specific areas, conformity to ASHA requirements is not seen.

In summary, then, how much and what kind of training is necessary to prepare competent speech-language pathologists interested in working in the school setting? Blanton suggested that such persons should have a background in anatomy and physiology. Current specifications for the CCC-SP are for training in the normal communication processes area, speech and language disorders, audiological assessment, and aural habilitation-rehabilitation. In addition, candidates for the CCC-SP must have 300 clock hours of specific clinical experiences. ASHA does not suggest that persons entering public school work must have student teaching experience, although many state certificates mandate such training. Coursework in related areas is required for the CCC-SP; the nature of such academic background is only suggested. Many states, on the other hand, require coursework in education and psychology; however, there appears to be little unanimity on what specific courses should be required. It is obvious that not all individuals, agencies, and certifying boards are in agreement as to how speech experts should be prepared for work in the public schools. And once such persons have been trained, there is also little agreement as to what to call them.

PROFESSIONAL TITLES

In the preface, a number of titles were used to refer to the individual who works with persons with communicative disorders. Included among those titles were speech teacher, speech correctionist, speech therapist, speech clinician, and speech-language pathologist; in the literature, other designations are found. From its outset, the profession of speech-language pathology has had some difficulty agreeing on the title its members should assume. *Speech teacher* evolved logically since classroom teachers originally assumed the role of the teacher of speech. Clearly, its application today is inappropriate even though it would not be surprising to hear it still being used in the school setting. Perhaps even some specialists employed in the public schools refer to themselves by that title. *Speech correctionist* was a title that appeared to emerge rather early in the development of the profession (circa 1900). At that time, its use may have been quite descriptive, since professionals were dealing with the correction of fluency, vocal, and articulatory problems. Currently, however, members of the profession have responsibilities far greater than the correction of those problems; use of *speech correctionist,* therefore, appears to be antiquated. Many individuals refer to themselves as *speech therapists*; besides the fact that the language component of the profession is omitted by this designation, the term *therapist* often carries the connotation that the professional is working under the direction of a physician. For example, physical and occupational therapists usually perform services under the supervision of a medical person. However, that is not necessarily true of speech and language professionals. Terms with some popularity today are *speech clinician* or *speech and language clinician.* As Van Hattum (1969) points out, this does not indicate that individuals are functioning within a clinical setting, but that rather they are functioning in a clinical manner. There are those, however, who feel that the title is too specific.

In 1962, the problem of a title for the profession was addressed by the ASHA Executive Council. Although it was acknowledged that some members of the profession were not concerned about the diversity of titles in use at that time, the Council studied the issue at some length (American Speech and Hearing Association Executive Council, 1962). They suggested that the public does not understand the role of the speech-language pathologist. The Council (1962) further stated,

Occasionally we discover that our image is somewhat out of focus. We don't attempt to ask the public to speak our name, for we have yet to give it to them. Until we do get a name, the condition of our absent or distorted image will remain. (p. 199)

Following a discussion of the importance of assuming an identity for the profession, the Council suggested the name should meet several criteria. Among these were that the title be a single word which would describe the total activities of its members and that the title could be easily written and spoken. Equally concerned with a name for the profession was Wendell Johnson, one of whose concerns was the inadequacy of the terms *speech pathology* and *audiology*. According to Johnson (1968), the separation of speech pathology and audiology suggested a division that should not occur, since these two areas of study are both related to oral communication. Johnson deemed it necessary to give the profession a single name and he, along with others, suggested *communicology*. Such a term would encourage unity rather than diversity among the members of the profession. Those involved in the field of communicology would be called *communicologists*. A review of current literature indicates, however, that Johnson's suggestion of a name for the profession was not taken up by the membership.

Although it was important to be aware of the various titles used by speech, language, and hearing specialists, the concern of this book is with the speech and language specialist in the school setting. Two surveys attempted to determine (1) what title or certificate designations were being used by the certifying agencies at the state level, (2) what certificate designations were thought to be used at the state level by practicing speech-language pathologists, and (3) which title the latter preferred. The first survey was distributed to state departments of education, and 92 percent of the states responded (Taylor, 1980). Table 1-1 lists the certificate designations reported by the various states and the number of states reporting each title. Professional titles and frequency data are also presented in Table 1-1.

Hahn (1980) mailed a questionnaire to 150 speech-language pathologists working in the school setting; 45 ASHA certified persons and 15 non-ASHA certified individuals responded to the survey. Among the questions posed were "What professional title or certificate designation is utilized in your state?" and "By what title do you prefer to be called?" Table 1-2 shows the responses to the first question.

Of those responding to this question, 22 indicated that the professional title employed in their states was *speech and language pathologist*. Yet only one state uses that designation on the official certificate and just four states use this title; it is therefore apparent that the data are skewed or inaccurate.

When asked which title they preferred, respondents replied as indicated in Table 1-2.

Table 1-1
Survey of Certificate Designations
and Professional Titles
Used by State Education Agencies

	No. of States
Certificate designation	
Speech correctionist	4
Basic speech and language	1
Standard speech and language	1
Speech pathology—Level 1	1
Speech pathology—Level 2	1
Speech and language impaired	1
Speech and communication disorders	1
Basic speech handicapped	1
Standard speech handicapped	1
Speech and hearing	1
Speech and hearing therapy	1
Speech disorders	1
Speech and language pathology	1
Speech and language	1
Professional title	
Speech and language clinician	4
Speech pathologist	4
Speech and language pathologist	4
Speech correctionist	3
Communication disorders specialist	3
Speech and hearing therapist	2
Speech and hearing clinician	2
Speech clinician	2
Speech correctionist/language specialist	1
Teacher of the speech handicapped	1
Teacher of the speech and hearing impaired	1
Language clinician	1
Speech and hearing teacher—therapist	1
School speech and hearing clinician	1
Speech therapist	1
Speech, language, and hearing therapist	1
Speech and hearing specialist	1

It is disturbing to realize that persons throughout the United States employ a variety of titles to refer to themselves and that certifying agencies utilize a similar diversity of titles and certificate designations. Even more amazing is that within a single state, various titles may be used. On December 7, 1979, the Southern Illinois University Placement Service Bulletin (1979)

Table 1-2

Survey of Professional Titles
Used by Speech-Language Pathologists

	No. of Responses[a]
Title or certificate designation used by state	
Speech and language pathologist	22
Speech therapist	12
Speech and language clinician	11
Speech pathologist	9
Speech and hearing therapist	7
Speech clinician	7
Speech correctionist	6
Communication disorders specialist	6
Speech and hearing clinician	3
Teacher of the speech and hearing impaired	3
Speech, language, and hearing clinician	3
Speech-language-hearing specialist	2
Language clinician	2
Speech and hearing specialist	2
Speech and language teacher/clinician	1
Teacher of the speech and hearing handicapped	1
Title preferred by respondents	
Speech and language pathologist	24
Speech and language clinician	13
Speech pathologist	7
Speech therapist	6
Communication disorders specialist	5
Speech-language therapist	4
Communication specialist	4
Speech correctionist	2
Speech and hearing therapist	2
Speech clinician	2
Language clinician	2
Speech, language, and hearing clinician	1
Speech and hearing specialist	1
Speech, language, and hearing pathologist	1
Teacher of the speech and hearing handicapped	1

SOURCE: Data from Hahn, 1980.
[a]Some respondents gave multiple answers.

listed the following vacancies for public school positions within the state: speech and language therapist, speech therapist, speech correctionist, speech-language pathologist, speech clinician, speech pathologist, and itinerant speech therapist. The official certificate of the state of Illinois is in "Speech and language impaired" and the designation given the holder of that certificate is *speech and language clinician* (State Board of Education, 1979). Yet not one of the positions described carried the title of *speech and language clinician*.

For a time, it appeared as if the problem of assigning a title to the speech and language specialist was over; in 1976, ASHA officially endorsed the title of *speech-language pathologist* (Healey & Dublinske, 1977). The Association hoped that the adoption of this title would end the confusion created by the numerous titles used by members of the profession both in schools and other professional settings. That hope has not materialized. Even today, university curricula continue to include coursework designed to prepare speech, language, and hearing clinicians, speech pathologists, speech clinicians, speech and language specialists, and public school clinicians. The terms "speech clinician," "speech-language clinician," and "speech pathologist" continue to be seen in the professional journals; similar terms can be heard at a convention of the American Speech-Language-Hearing Association. For better or for worse, then, the profession has failed to accept a single title. Moreover, reviewing the criteria suggested in 1962, the title currently used most often is not appropriate either. The Legislative Council indicated that the title (1) should be a single word, (2) should describe all professional activities, and (3) should be easily written and spoken. *Speech-language pathologist* meets just one of these criteria.

Although professionals within the field may be able to utilize various titles and understand they all relate to the same group of individuals, the public may not be so adept. One of the reasons that *speech-language pathologist* was adopted as the official title was that it best reflected the training and education of its members and the services delivered to communicatively disordered individuals (Healey & Dublinske, 1977). The consistent use of this title throughout the remainder of the book does not necessarily imply agreement with the designation. This title might be a little cumbersome in the public school setting, but it is employed because it has been recommended for use in all regulations surrounding Public Law (PL) 94-142.

REFERENCES

American Speech and Hearing Association Executive Council. A name for the profession of speech and hearing. *Asha,* 1962, *4,* 199–203.
Black, M. E. The origins and status of speech therapy in the schools. *Asha,* 1966, *8,* 419–425.

Eldridge, M. *A history of the treatment of speech disorders.* Edinburgh: Churchill Livingstone, 1968.

Hahn, C. *An investigation into current procedures of case finding, case selection and scheduling in the schools.* Unpublished M.S. thesis, Southern Illinois University at Edwardsville, 1980.

Haines, H. H. Trends in public school speech therapy. *Asha,* 1965, *7,* 187–190.

Healey, W. C., & Dublinske, S. Notes from the school services program. Official title: Speech-language pathologist. *Language, Speech, and Hearing Services in Schools,* 1977, *8,* 67.

Irwin, R. B. Speech and hearing therapy in the public schools of Ohio. *Journal of Speech and Hearing Disorders,* 1949, *14,* 63–68.

Johnson, W. Communicology? *Asha,* 1968, *10,* 43–56.

Moore, P., & Kester, D. G. Historical notes on speech correction in the pre-association era. *Journal of Speech and Hearing Disorders,* 1953, *18,* 48–53.

Southern Illinois University Placement Service Bulletin, 10, 1979.

State Board of Education, Illinois Office of Education. *Rules and regulations to govern the administration and operation of special education,* Springfield, 1979.

Taylor, J. S. Public school certification standards: Are they standard? *Asha,* 1980, *22,* 159–165.

Van Hattum, R. J. *Clinical speech in the schools.* Springfield, Illinois: Charles C Thomas, 1969.

2

The Communicatively Disordered Child and PL 94-142

The issue of a person's right to speech, language, and audiological services is a complex one—one with which we must come to grips. Not all communicatively handicapped children are being served by the public school, and I suggest that these children do have a right to such service. (Caccamo, 1974, p. 175)

The implementation of Public Law 94-142, Education for All Handicapped Children Act of 1975, has been heralded by many as signifying the end of a silent revolution on behalf of handicapped children in the United States. Actually, the educational rights of such individuals have been acknowledged in a steady progression of state and federal legislation throughout the years. The concept of free public education, for example, can be traced back as far as 1837; at that time, Massachusetts created a state board to oversee the education of children (Melcher, 1976). Provisions for the education of handicapped children were not in evidence, however, until 1911, when New Jersey created a statute that established such provisions. Other states providing education to the handicapped prior to the 1920s included Minnesota, Wisconsin, Illinois, and New York. A more recent example of state recognition of the needs of the handicapped is the landmark decision in *Pennsylvania Association for Retarded Children* v. *the Commonwealth of Pennsylvania.*

Although education has been considered an obligation of individual states, the federal government has been instrumental in obtaining rights for handicapped children and adults. By means of public laws, Congress has encouraged the construction of facilities for the retarded (PL 88-164), provided financial assistance to local education agencies (PL 89-10), and allocated funds for the education of handicapped children (PL 89-750). Each of these laws appears to have had some role in the development of PL 94-142.

STATE PARTICIPATION IN EDUCATION
FOR THE HANDICAPPED

The case of *Pennsylvania Association for Retarded Children* v. *the Commonwealth of Pennsylvania* is regarded as critical with regard to the education of handicapped children. In this instance, the School Code of the state was challenged and found to be unacceptable. On January 7, 1971, 13 retarded children, along with members of the Pennsylvania Association for Retarded Children (PARC), appeared in the federal district court; their initial goal was to obtain access to free education (Gilhool, 1973). Although the commonwealth provided education to exceptional children, a loophole in the law allowed for the exclusion of individuals with a mental age (MA) lower than five years. Actually, the education of such a child was "postponed" until an MA of five years was reached; in effect, this meant that a severely retarded child who would never achieve an MA of five would never receive public education. Therefore, the first concern in the PARC case was access to free public education.

A second goal was to ensure that the child received an education and that both parents and children played a role in determining the nature and quality of that training. What was being sought was justification for placing a child in a specific program, justification for maintaining the child in that program, and/or justification for changing a child's placement. Further, opportunities for parent and child participation in these decision-making processes were requested.

After hearing the testimony of a variety of witnesses, the commonwealth apparently acknowledged that a more adequate method of meeting the needs of its exceptional children must be found. Through a series of court orders and injunctions, modifications designed to improve the education of handicapped individuals in Pennsylvania were recommended.

Several patterns of reform are exemplified by the PARC decree (Kuriloff, True, Kirp, & Buss, 1974). Access to a free public education for mentally retarded children was mandated, and the identification of children excluded from schools was specified. Comprehensive evaluation of children already identified as retarded and of those previously excluded from public education was required. These procedures were designed to ensure that each child was accurately diagnosed and placed. Similarly, biannual reevaluations of all handicapped children were mandated, and due process hearings were made accessible to parents who questioned the accuracy of the diagnosis or the suitability of their child's educational placement. Finally, the decree addressed the issue of appropriate placement; although the *least restrictive environment* designation was not employed, that concept was described. Significant in the rulings was the stipulation that school officials must be able to justify the placement of children in specific educational programs.

In an attempt to assess the success of Pennsylvania's implementation of the decree in the PARC case, the Project on Student Classification and the Law (at the University of Pennsylvania) studied the critical issues (Kuriloff et al., 1974). Some of the findings of this project are included in this discussion, since many of the recommendations from the PARC decision resemble those of PL 94-142.

To comply with the initial recommendation that all children who had been excluded from free public education be identified and located, the Commonwealth Plan for Identification, Location and Evaluation of Mentally Retarded Children (COMPILE) was established. COMPILE publicized the search for retarded children extensively, and its efforts were supplemented by "Operation Childhunt," conducted by PARC. The target date for identification, evaluation, and placement of the excluded children was September 1972, only four months after authorization for the childfind was granted. Because of the time needed to secure additional personnel to evaluate the children, extreme burdens were placed on those districts attempting to comply with COMPILE's specifications. Further difficulties were encountered in the childfind when some districts apparently resisted the efforts. Despite these problems, it was generally agreed that the identification process was successful.

Evaluative procedures presented difficulties, owing, in part, to the large numbers of children requiring assessment and in part to the inappropriateness of the testing tool. The demands of initial testing and reevaluation eventually led the psychologists charged with these responsibilities to make the best of a difficult situation. In some cases, this included placing children on the basis of identification only. According to Kuriloff et al. (1974), review of the evaluation procedures was undertaken after these problems were encountered.

Difficulties were also encountered with the placements of retarded children. The consent agreement mandated that appropriate education, conducted by properly trained teachers, be provided to such children. Although the Commonwealth Plan to Educate and Train Mentally Retarded Children (COMPET) was developed, it did not meet the requirements established in that agreement. Later attempts to revise the plan were also unsuccessful. As of 1974, problems in the placement of retarded children in appropriate programs continued to be apparent.

With regard to the due process requirements of the decree, the Pennsylvania Right to Education Office was established. Among the responsibilities of this office were the supervision of due process hearings, the assignment of hearing officers, and the maintenance of records. Limited by insufficient staff, the Office had difficulty in executing all of its responsibilities. Assessing the role of the Office in due process hearings, it was apparent that confusion had been created by a lack of definition of terms. Since "appropriate placement" did not provide specific definitions of terms, the hearing officers used varying interpretations as they made their decisions. As a result, both the parents requesting a change of placement and school officials attempting to justify placement were confused. For the Office to be maximally effective, clarification of definitions was needed.

Although total compliance with the recommendation in *Pennsylvania Association for Retarded Children* v. *the Commonwealth of Pennsylvania* was not evident, significant changes in the educational management of retarded children were brought about. As indicated previously, the right to education irrespective of mental age was established, childfind procedures were implemented, and innovative programming designed to meet the needs of retarded children was initiated. Finally, despite the variations that existed in the due process hearings, parents become active participants in the educational planning for their children.

A similar decision was reached in the *Mills* v. *Board of Education of the District of Columbia* case of 1972 (Abeson & Zettel, 1977). In this instance, a class action suit on behalf of all handicapped children was initiated by the parents and guardians of seven District of Columbia children. The Mills decision concluded with a court order assuring all handicapped children the right to an appropriate, free public education.

The right of handicapped children to education has been reinforced by the passage of a number of state statutes and regulations. By 1972, 70 percent of the states had reportedly adopted legislation requiring the education of children with handicaps, as defined by each state's policy (Abeson & Zettel, 1977). Three years later, all but two states required the education of the majority of its handicapped children and, by 1977, only one state had not enacted such legislation.

It is apparent, then, that legislation at the state level contributed to a recognition of the rights of handicapped children. Parents were sometimes instrumental in bringing the issue into focus, as were special interest groups. Supplementary pressure has also been exerted in the form of federal legislation.

FEDERAL PARTICIPATION IN EDUCATION
FOR THE HANDICAPPED PRIOR TO PL 94-142

PL 88-164

Throughout the years, the federal government has provided incentives to the states with regard to the management of handicapped children. In 1963, Public Law 88-164, titled the Mental Retardation Facilities and Community Health Centers Construction Act of 1963 was enacted. Title I of this law appropriated funds

for project grants to assist in meeting the costs of construction of facilities for research, or research and related purposes, relating to human development, whether biological, medical, social, or behavioral, which may assist in finding the causes, and means of prevention of mental retardation, or in finding means of ameliorating the effects of mental retardation. (Public Law 88-164, 1963)

Part B of the law authorized appropriations for the construction of university-affiliated facilities for the retarded; such facilities were to provide services to the retarded as well as training to professional workers. Part C provided grants for the construction of public and nonprofit facilities for the mentally retarded. Finally, Title III dealt with the preparation of teachers of handicapped children. Fellowships, training grants, and traineeships were authorized to educate "speech correctionists" and teachers of the hard of hearing and deaf. This act, inspired by proposals to the Congress by President John F. Kennedy, not only provided incentives for the construction of facilities for the retarded, but also attempted to encourage the training of personnel to work with the handicapped (Hagerty & Howard, 1978).

PL 89-10

In 1965, PL 89-10, the Elementary and Secondary Education Act of 1965 was enacted. Title I provided financial assistance

to local educational agencies serving areas with concentration of children from low income families and to expand and improve their educational programs by various means (including preschool programs) which contribute particularly to meeting the special education needs of educationally deprived children. (Public Law 89-10, 1965)

According to Hagerty and Howard (1978), many administrators failed to take advantage of Title I even though programming for the handicapped was possible under this section.

Title II, School Library Resources, Textbooks, and Other Instructional Materials, required that individual states prepare plans for the acquisition of such materials. Although special resources for the handicapped could be requested in the state plan, little evidence exists to indicate that states sought such funding (Hagerty & Howard, 1978).

Supplementary educational centers and services were encouraged under Title III of PL 89-10; it was reported that some of the most innovative programs developed under this title were designed to assist the handicapped (Hagerty & Howard, 1978). A later revision of the law required that 15 percent of the available funds be allocated to programming for the handicapped. Title IV dealt with the authority of the Office of Education, and Title V of the act provided grants to strengthen state departments of education. Under the latter section, states could provide local educational agencies with consultative and technical assistance, as well as services related to a variety of areas including the education of the handicapped.

PL 89-750

On November 3, 1966, Public Law 89-750, Elementary and Secondary Education Amendments of 1966, was enacted; the most significant amendment was Title VI of the act, Education of Handicapped Children. The purpose of Title VI was to provide grants

for the purpose of assisting the states in the initiation, expansion, and improvement of programs and projects (including the acquisition of equipment and where necessary the construction of school facilities) for the education of handicapped children (as defined in section 602) at the preschool, elementary and secondary school levels. (Public Law 89-750, 1966)

Section 602 defined "handicapped children" and included the hard of hearing, deaf, and speech impaired. In order to receive funding, individual states were required to submit plans to the Commissioner of Education; eleven criteria were employed to evaluate the state plans. Finally, Title VI established a National Advisory Committee on Handicapped Children and the Bureau for the Education and Training of the Handicapped.

PL 91-230

Additional bills were passed by Congress on behalf of the handicapped. Public Law 91-230, and extension of the Elementary and Secondary Education Act of 1965, was enacted on April 13, 1970 (Public Law 91-230, 1970). Title VI of that bill codified much of the previously passed legislation (Hagerty & Howard, 1978). In addition to the provisions established in Title VI of PL 89-750, PL 91-230 authorized funding for the development of centers and services to meet the special needs of the handicapped, for the training of personnel for the education of the handicapped (including "speech correctionists"), for research in the education of the handicapped, and for the development of instructional media for the handicapped and special programs for children with specific learning disabilities.

PL 93-112

The purpose of Section 504 of PL 93-112, The Rehabilitation Act of 1973, is to terminate discrimination against handicapped individuals. Specifically, Section 504 provides that

no otherwise qualified handicapped individual in the United States shall, solely by reason of his handicap, be excluded from participation in, be denied the benefits of or be subjected to discrimination under any program or activity receiving federal financial assistance. (Public Law 93-112, 1973)

A civil rights statute, Section 504 contains six parts. Subpart *A* is concerned with general provisions, *B* with employment practices, *C* with program accessibility, *E* with postsecondary education, *F* with health, welfare, and social services, and *G* with procedures. Subpart *D* considers the education of preschool, elementary, and secondary school-age handicapped children. The provisions of this part of the act resemble those of the more recent PL 94-142.

They require basically, that recipients operating public education programs provide a free appropriate education to each qualified handicapped child in the most normal setting appropriate. The regulation also sets forth evaluation requirements designed to ensure the proper classification and placement of handicapped children, and due process procedures for resolving disputes over placement of students. While the Department does not intend to review individual placement decisions, it does intend to ensure that testing and evaluation procedures required by the regulation are carried out, and that school systems provide an adequate opportunity for parents to challenge and seek review of these critical decisions. (Public Law 93-112, 1973)

PL 93-380

In 1974, Public Law 93-380, Education Amendments of 1974, was enacted. Among the significant sections of the Act was Section 513, known popularly as the Buckley Amendment or the Family Educational Rights and Privacy Act of 1974. Part a, 1 dealt with the rights of parents "to inspect and review any and all official records, files, and data directly related to their children" (Public Law 93-380, 1974). Further, Part a, 2 provided the opportunity for parents to request a hearing

to challenge the content of their child's school records, and to ensure that the records are not inaccurate, misleading, or otherwise in violation of the privacy or other rights of students, and to provide an opportunity for the correction or deletion of any such inaccurate, misleading, or otherwise inappropriate data contained therein. (Public Law 93-380, 1974)

Section 438 also prohibited the release of confidential information without the written permission of the parents.

Sections 611–621 specifically addressed the education of the handicapped and offered financial assistance to the states in developing complete educational programming at the preschool, elementary school, and secondary school levels; the appropriations were applicable to the fiscal year 1975. The rights of parents and children with regard to due process were emphasized in Section 612, as was the concept of least restrictive environment. The law required the states to ensure that

to the maximum extent appropriate, handicapped children including children in public or private institutions or other care facilities are educated with children who are not handicapped, and that special classes, separate schooling, or other removal of handicapped children from the regular education environment occurs only when the nature or severity of the handicap is such that education in regular classes with the use of supplementary aids and services cannot be achieved satisfactorily. (Public Law 93-380, 1974)

Finally, the Act required that the states formulate a plan for meeting the needs of all handicapped children and establish a time frame for implementing the plan.

It is apparent, therefore, that concern for the education of handicapped children evolved over a period of years and that this concern was reflected in the enactment of various public laws. Initially, the federal government provided financial assistance for the construction of facilities for the mentally retarded and encouraged research into the problems experienced by this population. Early legislation allocated funding for the training of personnel to work with the handicapped and for the development of specific programming. Later public laws concerned the rights of parents and their handicapped children to participate in educational planning and encouraged placement of children in the least restrictive environment. All of this legislation paved the way for the most significant law with regard to the handicapped, PL 94-142.

PUBLIC LAW 94-142

Purpose

Preparatory to stating the purpose of PL 94-142 in the official document, several facts related to the development of the law were presented. Section 3 stated that more than eight million handicapped children were living in the United States in 1975, and that the needs of these children were not being met. Further, the majority of these individuals were not receiving appropriate education, and one million children were excluded entirely from education with their peers. The document also stated that many children had unidentified handicaps that limited their success in school and that some children with detected handicaps were forced to receive services from outside agencies because their needs could not be met in the public school setting. Assuming that, given appropriate financial assistance, local and state educational agencies could provide services to handicapped children and that it was the responsibility of these agencies to provide such services, the federal government concluded that it was in the best interest of the nation to provide financial assistance to state and local educational agencies so that they could implement programs for the handicapped and assure such individuals equal protection under the law. The purpose, then, of PL 94-142 was presented as follows:

> It is the purpose of this Act to assure that all handicapped children have available to them...a free appropriate education which emphasizes special education and related services designed to meet their unique needs, to assure that the rights of handicapped children and their parents or guardians are protected, to assist states and localities to provide for the education of all handicapped children, and to assess and assure the effectiveness of efforts to educate handicapped children. (Public Law 94-142, 1975)

Definitions

In order to identify the target population and the types of services which must be provided, Section 602 included definitions of handicaps covered by the law. Among the children identified as handicapped were those who are hard of hearing, deaf, and speech impaired. The hard of hearing child is one whose impairment affects his ability to function in the classroom. Deaf children are those whose hearing is nonfunctional in the school setting. Speech impaired children have disorders of fluency, language, articulation, and/or voice that adversely affect their performances in the classroom.

"Special education" is defined as "classroom instruction, instruction in physical education, home instruction, and instruction in hospitals and institutions"; such education must be designed to meet the unique needs of the individual child (Public Law 94-142, 1975). Related services include transportation and supportive services (including speech pathology and audiology) required by each child in order to benefit from the special education services (an interpretation of this aspect of the law is presented later in the chapter). Medical services for diagnostic purposes are also designated as supportive. Another important requirement defined by the law is the *individualized education program* (IEP). Although Chapter 6 addresses IEPs at length, the following definition should provide a preliminary understanding of the intent of this requirement.

The term "individualized education program" means a written statement for each handicapped child developed in any meeting by a representative of the local educational agency or an intermediate educational unit who shall be qualified to provide, or supervise the provision of, specially designed instruction to meet the unique needs of handicapped children, the teacher, the parents or guardian of such child, and, whenever appropriate, such child, which statement shall include (A) a statement of the present levels of educational performance of such child, (B) a statement of annual goals, including short-term instructional objectives, (C) a statement of the specific educational services to be provided to such child, and the extent to which such child will be able to participate in regular educational programs, (D) the projected date for initiation and anticipated duration of such services, and (E) appropriate objective criteria and evaluation procedures and schedules for determining, on at least an annual basis, whether instructional objectives are being achieved. (Public Law 94-142, 1975)

Entitlements and Allocations

Although a lengthy discussion of entitlements and allocations is not appropriate in a text of this kind, some aspects of these portions of the law require attention. Essentially, the law allocates funds to each state based on the number of handicapped children between the ages of 3 and 21 who are receiving special education and related services. An average of the number of individuals receiving such services on specific dates each year determines the official count. The funding formula is based on a percentage of the excess cost of educating a handicapped student in terms of average per-pupil expenditure. In 1978, the law authorized 5 percent of the expenditure multiplied by the total number of handicapped children receiving services; that percentage was to increase to 10 percent in 1979, 20 percent in 1980, and 30 percent in 1981. Beginning in 1982, and continuing each year thereafter, 40 percent of the average per-pupil expenditure may be authorized. It should be noted that the law will permit allocation of funds for no more than 12 percent of the school age population. PL 94-142 allows the states to retain 25 percent of the appropriated funding for administrative purposes and supportive services, with the remainder being distributed to the local educational agencies. No more than five percent of the total may be used for administrative costs at the state level. In terms of dollars and cents, then, it is apparent that individual states and local educational agencies must be accurate in determining the number of children receiving special education and related services so they may benefit fully from federal allocations.

Eligibility

In order to be eligible for federal assistance, the state must show that it has a policy that "assures all handicapped children the right to a free public education" (Public Law 94-142, 1975). Each state must have developed a plan designed to provide complete educational opportunities to all handi-capped children. This plan must include a timetable for achieving that goal and a description of the necessary facilities, personnel, and services. Educa-tional programming must be available for all handicapped children between the ages of 3 and 21 by September 1980 (by September 1978 for children be-tween 3 and 18) "unless the application of such requirements would be incon-sistent with state law or practice" (Public Law 94-142, 1975). Further, the state must have developed procedures for locating and evaluating children in need of special programming. The plan must also conform to priorities specified in PL 94-142 for providing special education to the handicapped. First priority is given to handicapped children who are not receiving an educa-tion; second priority is given to those severely handicapped children who are not receiving an adequate education. Additional eligibility requirements are that (1) the local education agency maintain IEPs for each handicapped child, (2) handicapped children be educated with nonhandicapped children whenever possible, and (3) evaluative procedures be nonbiased with respect to race or culture. Regarding the third requirement, it is mandated that pro-cedures be provided in the child's native language; further, more than one evaluative instrument or procedure must be utilized. "The provision, in ef-fect, orders that assessment procedures be multi-factored, multi-sourced, and carried out by qualified personnel" (Ballard & Zettel, 1977, p. 184).

Procedural Safeguards

Section 615 of PL 94-142 requires that all states and local educational agencies receiving assistance assure that handicapped children and their parents are "guaranteed procedural safeguards with respect to the provision of free appropriate education" (Public Law 94-142, 1975). The agencies are required to permit parents or guardians of handicapped children to have ac-cess to all relevant records "with respect to the identification, evaluation, and educational placement of the child" (Public Law 94-142, 1975). Parents or guardians must also have the opportunity to request an independent evalua-tion of the child. Surrogates must be appointed to represent the child whose parents or guardians are unknown or unavailable. Additional safeguards re-quire that parents be informed in writing whenever a change in their child's program is proposed or when the agency refuses to initiate a change in that program. Parents must also be given an opportunity to object to any aspect of the child's educational management.

If parents question the educational opportunities available to their child, they must have access to an impartial due process hearing to be conducted by the local, intermediate, or state educational agency. When the hearing is held at the local or intermediate level, appeals may be made to the state educa-tional agency; subsequent appeals may be taken to the state or federal courts.

With regard to the hearing itself, all parties must be allowed to be accompanied and advised by counsel or by individuals knowledgeable about handicapped children. Any party may present evidence, cross-examine, and/or request the attendance of witnesses. Written or electronic records of the proceedings, findings, and decision of the hearing must be made available to all parties.

Although other sections of PL 94-142 consider additional aspects of the law, this discussion has been limited to those parts that should be of interest to speech-language pathologists. Before discussing the implications of PL 94-142 and Section 504 for speech-language pathologists, let us consider the laws as they have been upheld in the courts.

Implementation of PL 94-142 and Section 504

As noted earlier, litigation played a large role in the development of both state and federal legislation designed to protect the educational rights of handicapped children. Since the enactment of the laws discussed, the requirements and due process provisions have been tested. The following cases illustrate the impact that both acts have had on the rights of handicapped citizens; all cases were reported by the Federal Programs Advisory Service and published in the *Handicapped Requirements Handbook* (Federal Advisory Service, 1979).

In the *Mattie T.* v. *Holladay* case, officials of the Mississippi Department of Education were charged with failing "to adopt sufficient policies and procedures to ensure the plaintiff's procedural safeguards under the Education for All Handicapped Children Act (Federal Advisory Service, 1979, p. iv: A:xxviii). The court ordered state officials to develop a plan to comply with PL 94-142. It further affirmed the right to an appropriate education as stated in Section 504 of the Rehabilitation Act of 1973. In this decision, PL 94-142 was employed to require that Mississippi implement a plan for compliance with the law.

The North Carolina Association for Retarded Children brought a class action suit against the State of North Carolina Board of Education in 1978. The Association alleged that residents of four mental institutions were denied access to free public education because they were retarded; this was in violation of PL 94-142 and Section 504. A consent agreement reached in July 1978 provided for location of all mentally retarded children in need of free and appropriate educational opportunities. A citizens' advocacy program was also established.

In the *Frederich L.* v. *Thomas* case, 1977, the plaintiff, a learning disabled child, sued the School District of Philadelphia. It was alleged that the district did not provide appropriate education for learning disabled children. As a result of the findings of the case, the district was ordered to locate all learning disabled children.

The concept of education in the least restrictive environment was tested in the *Hairston* v. *Drosick* case. The parents of a spina bifida child contested the school's decision that the child could not be placed in the regular classroom unless the mother accompanied her. (School officials had recommended homebound instruction or placement in a classroom for the physically handicapped.) Violation of Section 504 was claimed by the plaintiff. The court ruled that a minimally handicapped child could not be excluded from the regular classroom without a "bona fide educational reason" and concurred that the child's exclusion was a violation of Section 504.

A recent Gallup poll dealt with the public's attitude toward this same concept (Gallup, 1979). The first question asked was whether the respondents felt that mentally handicapped students should be educated in the same classrooms with "normal" students or placed in special classrooms. Of the individuals questioned, 77 percent indicated that special classroom placement was preferable. Only 13 percent felt that mentally handicapped students should be educated with "normal" students and the remaining 10 percent had no opinion. When asked whether physically handicapped children should be placed in special classes, only 36 percent responded affirmatively. The majority of respondents (53 percent) felt that they should be placed with other students, and 11 percent had no opinion.

The 1979 case of *Larry P.* v. *Riles* involved violations of Title VI of the Civil Rights Act of 1964, the Education of All Handicapped Children Act, and Section 504 of the Rehabilitation Act of 1973 (Federal Advisory Service, 1979). The plaintiffs in the case represented a group of black students in California placed in classes for the educable mentally retarded. The plaintiffs alleged that the tests used as the basis for placement were culturally biased. The court ruled that the rights of the plaintiffs had indeed been violated. It found that the

defendents have utilized standardized intelligence tests that are racially and culturally biased, have a discriminatory impact on black children, and have not been validated for the purpose of essentially permanent placement of black children into educationally dead end, isolated, and stigmatized classes for the so-called educable mentally retarded. (Federal Advisory Service, 1979, p. iv:A:xli)

The involvement of a speech-language pathologist in a PL 94-142 dispute was reported in 1980 (Miller, Miller, & Madison, 1980). In this case, the parents of a 16-year-old deaf student questioned the management of their son, specifically his placement and individualized education program. With regard to speech-language intervention, the parents maintained that the youngster was receiving insufficient therapy. Although the final decision was favorable to the school district, the rights of parents to object to treatment plans are exemplified in this case. Additional reports of due process decisions involving speech-language pathologists were presented by Dublinske (1980).

In one case, academic summer programming for a language disordered child was sought and obtained; similar decisions have been made in several states. In another case, the request of the parents of a first-grade hearing impaired child to have the school district provide an interpreter was denied. The Commissioner of Education (New York Education Department) found that the child was progressing satisfactorily without such assistance, and the parents were unable to provide documentation to the contrary.

This brief discussion suggests that parents and advocacy groups are becoming cognizant of the various laws and regulations governing the educational rights of the handicapped and are taking advantage of them. Speech-language pathologists, as involved professionals, must be conversant with relevant legislation and its impact on the clients they serve.

THE IMPLICATIONS OF STATE AND FEDERAL LEGISLATION FOR SCHOOL SPEECH-LANGUAGE PATHOLOGISTS

Although the passage of legislation at the state and federal levels should have been greeted with enthusiasm by all professionals involved with handicapped children, there is no doubt that difficulties in interpretation and implementation have tempered this enthusiasm. A perusal of the literature revealed one offering entitled "Staying out of jail," an article dealing with the IEP requirements of PL 94-142 (Reynolds, 1978). This title may reflect the attitude with which some professionals are approaching current regulations. As the September 1978 deadline for implementation of PL 94-142 approached, some anxiety was apparent among speech-language pathologists. Most, however, realized that much of what was required by the law had always been done by conscientious speech-language pathologists. Additionally, they realized that state and local requirements regarding the law were sometimes more involved than the federal law itself.

The Impact of State Legislation: Massachusetts

As mentioned earlier, the majority of states have enacted legislation to protect the rights of handicapped children. Blanchard and Nober (1978) reported on Massachusetts Law Chapter 766 and the effect it has had on school speech-language pathologists; their report is summarized in the following discussion as an example of the impact legislation may have on the functioning of professionals in the school setting.

The commonwealth of Massachusetts was among the first to enact comprehensive legislation with reference to education. According to Blanchard and Nober (1978), Special Education Chapter 766, passed in 1972, "assures that all handicapped children are offered a free, least restricting, appropriate public education; that the rights of handicapped children and parents are protected; and that states and localities provide these services'' (p. 77).*

The law was implemented in September 1974, and fourteen months later, a study was initiated to determine the effect that Chapter 766 had had on school speech-language pathologists. Employing a questionnaire format, Blanchard and Nober (1978) attempted to obtain the following data:

1. demographic information about the clinicians' case load numbers, number of speech, language, and hearing clinicians employed by the local school district, job status (full- or part-time), and present Core Evaluation Team role;
2. clinicians' perceptions of the importance of selected competency skills, pre-766 and current;
3. professional activity changes as a direct result of Chapter 766;
4. case-load profile changes;
5. clinicians' interest in future formal training in selected competency areas. (p. 78)

Respondents to the questionnaire were 211 people attending regional workshops. With regard to demographic data, it was determined that there was a 22 percent increase in the number of clinicians employed in the districts after the implementation of Chapter 766. Maximum case load (the number of children seen for therapy each week) was mandated by Chapter 766 to be 50. Before the implementation of the law, the average case load was 86.1. The average case load at the time of the survey was 53 children per week. As the majority (95 percent) of the clinicians were employed on a full-time basis, it was determined that districts were not employing part-time persons to meet the mandates of Chapter 766. Most clinicians in the state reported at least some involvement with the Core Evaluation Team; only 1 percent were not participating at the time of the survey.

To assess perceptions of the importance of various competency skills, the investigators asked clinicians to rate the importance of 35 skills, first using pre-766 judgments and then comparing these assessments with current perceptions. Included were identification (screening), evaluative, administrative, treatment, and educational skills.

The skills that increased most in perceived importance from pre-766 to the current time were (1) preschool screening, (2) kindergarten screening, (3) team screening, (4) writing of behavioral objectives, (5) preparation of educational plans, (6) service as a case manager, (7) team decision-making, (8) preschool intervention. (Blanchard & Nober, 1978, p. 79)

In responding to the item on modification of clinical activities as a result of 766, clinicians did not report a reduction in direct contact time (actual time

*From "The Impact of State and Federal Legislation on Public School Speech, Language, and Hearing Clinicians" by M. M. Blanchard and E. H. Nober. *Language, Speech, and Hearing Services in Schools,* 1978, *9,* 77–84. Reprinted by permission.

spent in therapy). This was apparently because of additional staff and reduced case loads. Clinicians reported increased involvement in interaction with other professionals and parents, in-service training, supervision, preschool screening, "case-load threshold testing," and preparation of materials and reports. With regard to case load distribution, the clinicians reported increases in the number of children who presented disorders of language and hearing, as well as those with multiple disorders and handicaps of organic etiology (Blanchard & Nober, 1978). The final item involved the interest of the clinicians in additional training. Listed in descending order of interest were language therapy, evaluative procedures, interpretation of test results from related disciplines, consultative skills, therapy for preschool and elementary school age children, auditory discrimination training, and execution of in-service training programs.

Because Massachusetts Law Chapter 766 and PL 94-142 are similar, this discussion of the effects of implementation of the former seems warranted. Speech-language pathologists in schools throughout the country may be experiencing similar modifications in their therapy programs as they comply with state and federal regulations.

The Impact of Federal Legislation

In addition to PL 94-142, the law receiving greatest attention in professional literature is PL 93-380, Section 513, Family Educational Rights and Privacy Act of 1974, also known, as mentioned earlier, as the Buckley Amendment. Enactment of this law allowed students and their parents the right to inspect information contained in all relevant official records concerning the students. In addition, it required schools to obtain the written permission of parents before student records could be released to any outside source. The law also limited the release of "any personally identifiable data on students and their families on the grounds that such actions constitute a violation of the right to privacy and confidentiality" (Healey, 1975, p. 115).

Initial concerns created by the law included the impact of the regulations on research (Healey, 1975). It was projected that research efforts might be hindered by the inaccessibility of such information. As the chair of an internal review board overseeing the participation of human subjects in research, the author concurs that some research efforts have been complicated by the Buckley Amendment. It should be pointed out, however, that researchers obtaining informed consent from subjects or their parents (in the case of minors) continue to be able to conduct sensitive and pertinent studies without violating Section 513. In retrospect, the concern with legislative impact on research proved to be unnecessary.

Another issue raised involved the inclusiveness of the term "official records." Healey questioned whether this included information collected by the speech-language pathologist. Pickering (1976) addressed the Buckley Amendment and the potential effect it might have on the records maintained by professionals in this area. She commented on the fact that speech-language pathologists have enjoyed the luxury of a closed system of record keeping. With the advent of the amendment, objectivity and accuracy in reporting are even more essential since parents and students have access to this information. Pickering (1976) concluded that "we must now ask ourselves to examine what we write as well as how well we write it. If we are not willing to let our clients and their parents see our records, perhaps we ought not be saying certain things at all" (p. 133).

Although some inconveniences may have resulted from enactment of the Buckley Amendment, there is little doubt that it is serving a necessary function. Speech-language pathologists involved in research should not be inhibited by the requirements of Section 513. Those investigators desiring to collect personal data for research purposes should be able to obtain informed consent if the project's objectives and procedures are presented to potential subjects (or their parents) in a reasonable manner.

With regard to accessibility of records, speech-language pathologists should maintain objective information on the clients they serve. The professional who declares that a child is "language disordered" without verifying objective data is suspect, but the speech-language pathologist who bases such a diagnosis on analysis of a language sample and the results of standardized language tests will have no concern about making these records accessible to parents. Therefore, this provision of the law should present no problem to the professional speech-language pathologist.

Questions regarding the impact of PL 94-142 were raised and answered by Dublinske and Healey (1978). Following presentation of the general principles of the law, the authors discussed terms relevant to the speech-language pathologist. In defining "deaf," "hard of hearing," and "speech impaired," the law specifies that the disorder "adversely affects educational performance." Does that mean that it must be demonstrated that a child with a vocal disorder—hypernasality, for example—is not performing well academically as a result of this problem before he qualifies as communicatively handicapped? According to Dublinske and Healey (1978), the answer to this question is negative: "Educational performance is not defined in the law or the regulation. However, educational performance has been interpreted broadly to include not only academic performance but also a child's social and emotional performance, and interpersonal relationships" (p. 190).*

This interpretation allows for children with fluency or vocal disorders to

---

*From "Questions and Answers for the Speech-Language Pathologist and Audiologist" by S. Dublinske and W. C. Healey. *Asha,* 1978, *20,* 188–205. Reprinted by permission.

receive services even though their communicative disorders may not affect academic performance.

Another issue addressed by Dublinske and Healey concerned language impaired children. These children are included in the definition of "speech impaired" but are also cited in references to children with "specific learning disabilities." The fact that such students are included in both areas does not preclude the provision of services by speech-language pathologists.

Under PL 94-142, the speech-language pathologist provides the following services:

1. Identification of children with speech or language disorders.
2. Diagnosis and appraisal of specific speech or language disorders.
3. Referral for medical or other professional attention necessary for the habilitation of speech or language disorders.
4. Provision of speech and language services for the habilitation or prevention of communicative disorders.
5. Counseling and guidance of parents, children, and teachers regarding speech and language disorders. (Dublinske & Healey, 1978, p. 191)

Even the student-in-training is aware that the foregoing activities have always been considered among the responsibilities of the speech-language pathologist. In the school setting, the term *screening* has frequently been used to specify the identification process. Children are screened for disorders of articulation, voice, hearing, fluency, and language. After parental permission is secured, children who may present some problem are evaluated and considered for services. In some cases, referrals are made. Persons immediately concerned with the child—and, if appropriate, the child himself or herself—are advised of the diagnosis and the nature of the services to be provided. Counseling of these individuals is provided as therapy progresses. It is evident, then, that speech-language pathologists in the schools have been involved in all areas of service outlined in PL 94-142. The rigor with which some of the areas are pursued might be increased by the law but, in general, the responsibilities should be familiar ones to these professionals.

Earlier in the chapter, the nature of the service provided by speech-language pathologists was described. It appears that PL 94-142 includes speech pathology and audiology as related services rather than special education services. The latter term is defined as "specially designed instruction, at no cost to the parent, designed to meet the unique needs of a handicapped child, including classroom instruction, instruction in physical education, home instruction, and instruction in hospitals and institutions" (Public Law 94-142, 1975). According to Dublinske and Healey (1978),

The regulations indicate that the term includes speech-language pathology and many other services if they consist of specially designed instruction provided at no cost to the parents to meet the unique needs of a handicapped child and if considered "special education" rather than a "related service" under state standards. (p. 191)

Included as "related services" under the law are transportation and other support services including speech pathology and audiology. According to the law, children must be receiving special education services rather than related services in order to qualify for 94-142 funding. It would appear, then, that children with isolated communicative disorders would not be considered eligible for funding. Interpretation of the law does not confirm this, however. According to Dublinske and Healey, these definitions permit the inclusion of speech-language pathology and audiology services as both "special education" and "related services." To the child whose primary disability is in speech and language, "special education" in speech-language pathology is provided. "Related services" in speech-language pathology are appropriate for the child whose primary handicap is in an area such as mental retardation. Interpretation of the law suggests that the speech-language pathologist may provide either special education services or related services to communicatively disordered children; both types of services qualify for funding under PL 94-142.

Although Chapter 3 considers the assessment of communicatively disordered children in depth, some discussion of the impact of PL 94-142 on evaluative procedures is appropriate. First, the law mandates that children must be assessed before they may be placed in any type of special program. Further, the testing procedures must be nonbiased with regard to race or culture, they must be administered in the child's native language or "mode of communication" by a qualified professional, they must test what is purportedly tested, and they must take into account any disabilities that the child may have. There is little doubt that some of these qualifications might pose problems to the speech-language pathologists. Take, for example, the Peabody Picture Vocabulary Test (PPVT), a tool familiar to speech-language pathologists. Because this test was standardized on a group of white children in Tennessee, might it not be considered racially biased when used with black children? Further, many tests available to speech-language pathologists have questionable pertinence with regard to functional communicative ability; should this be taken into account in analyzing the results of such testing? In short, the assessment procedures recommended by PL 94-142 may be troublesome, but necessary.

Although the speech-language pathologist determines what evaluative tools and procedures should be utilized, it is necessary that a diagnosis be based on the results of more than one test. The child with an articulatory disorder would not be diagnosed as having such a problem on the basis of a conversational speech sample only; it would also be necessary to administer a standardized test of articulation. Similarly, a child could not be diagnosed as language disordered on the basis of the results of a vocabulary test.

It should be noted that parental consent is required before such an assessment is undertaken; the exception to this rule is parental failure to respond to a request for consent to an evaluation. In this case, several options may be available. According to Dublinske and Healey (1978), these include:

1. Compel the parents to respond through the due process hearing or court action.
2. Initiate the assessment after giving prior notice.
3. Retain the child in the present placement until consent is obtained.
4. Refuse placement of any kind until the issue is resolved. (p. 193)

Speech-language pathologists must be cognizant of the requirements regarding evaluation, as well as of steps that may be appropriate if the parents fail to agree to such an assessment.

One of the outstanding features of PL 94-142 is the mandate that handicapped children must be placed in the least restrictive environment. Actually, communicatively impaired children have been so placed for years. Most children remained in the regular classroom and were seen intermittently for speech-language therapy. This prototype of *mainstreaming* was not the result of farsightedness on the part of speech-language pathologists; rather it was due to a lack of placement opportunities for communicatively disordered children. This early therapy schedule might have been effective with children with isolated articulatory defects, but it did not meet the needs of children with serious language disorders. Today, it is recommended that a continuum of management alternatives be made available for all handicapped children. For students with language disorders, such alternatives might include placement in a special language classroom for the entire day, placement in such a class for a portion of the day, placement in the regular classroom with hour-long sessions in the resource room daily, or placement in the regular classroom with intermittent or intensive speech-language therapy delivered in the traditional manner. Additional information on the service continuum is contained in Chapter 4.

Considerable attention has been focused on the *individualized education program* (IEP) requirement of PL 94-142. Speech-language pathologists should have little difficulty complying with this stipulation of the law since professionals have been employing modified versions of IEPs for years. Specific information concerning the development and execution of IEPs is presented in Chapter 6.

One final aspect of PL 94-142 should be mentioned. A previous discussion of the funding schedule indicated that states in compliance would be eligible for up to 40 percent reimbursement of excess cost expenditures for handicapped children in 1982 and each year thereafter. The critical factor is that states must be in compliance; they must indeed be meeting all requirements of the law. According to Dublinske and Healey (1978), if parent or advocacy groups feel that a district or state receiving PL 94-142 funding is not in compliance, they may notify the state superintendent or commissioner of education, the regional HEW compliance officers, or a variety of other officials. "If the laws are going to be enforced, parents and advocacy organizations, such as speech and hearing associations, are going to have to alert authorities when noncompliance is observed (Dublinske & Healey, 1978, p. 205). Whether this method of notifying officials if districts are not in compliance is effective or not is questionable.

Recently, the author had a conversation with a speech-language pathologist working in a major midwestern city. It was reported by the professional that special educators in her district had not developed IEPs for the 1979–1980 year. It seems that during the summer of 1979, the chief administrative officer of the special education program had decided to revise the IEP format; he had not completed the revision by September, and so there was an initial delay in distributing the information. At some later point, the revised and printed forms were misplaced in a warehouse. Many superintendents and other school officials searched the warehouse unsuccessfully for the missing IEP forms. As the final one-third of the school year approached, the special educators were told that if they felt uncomfortable without IEPs, they should not work with the handicapped children. In an attempt to initiate action to rectify the situation, the speech-language pathologist contacted the state consultant and an official of the American Speech-Language-Hearing Association. In both instances, she was given sympathy but no hope of intervention.

In a situation similar to the one just described, a speech-language pathologist attempted to inform parents of their rights to due process. As the story goes, it was a building principal who reprimanded the speech-language pathologist for providing too much information to the parents. Clearly, noncompliance on the part of the local education agency was reflected in both situations.

DISCUSSION

State and federal legislation should serve to strengthen and improve the services provided by the speech-language pathologist and to provide opportunities not available previously. The child with a language disorder should be afforded a placement that meets his or her needs; this exemplifies a wider range of program alternatives. A reduction in case load should also result from implementation of PL 94-142; it is impossible to see 80 children weekly if each child requires 30 minutes of individual therapy each day. At the same time, speech-language pathologists may experience a modification in the time requirements of a public school position; participation in assessment activities, staffings, IEP conferences, and report writing claims more time than it did in the days before PL 94-142. In general, however, recent legislation should be viewed from a positive standpoint.

The final consideration must be the realities of the situation created by

PL 94-142. For example, many school districts do not have sufficient person-nel to provide appropriate services to all of the communicatively disordered children in that area. Reduced case loads were mentioned earlier as one of the positive results of PL 94-142; if a reduction in case load requires that a number of communicatively disordered children not be seen at all, then a violation of PL 94-142 occurs. Is it better to err on the side of providing some services to all children or appropriate services to a few? Most administrators would probably view the first option as preferable; most speech-language pathologists intent upon keeping their positions would concur. The extensive rights afforded parents in participating in their child's educational program have also created problems. Do parents always know what is best for their handicapped child, especially if that child presents an enigmatic disorder such as stuttering? These are areas of concerns for the speech-language pathologist with regard to the law; we may hope that future interpretations will provide answers to these concerns and put the finishing touches on the silent revolu-tion on behalf of handicapped children.

REFERENCES

Abeson, A., & Zettel, J. The end of the quiet revolution: The education for all handi-capped children act of 1975. *Exceptional Children,* 1977, *44,* 114–128.

Ballard, J., & Zettel, J. Public Law 94-142 and Section 504: What they say about rights and protections. *Exceptional Children,* 1977, *44,* 177–185.

Blanchard, M. M., & Nober, E. H. The impact of state and federal legislation on public school speech, language, and hearing clinicians. *Language, Speech, and Hearing Services in Schools,* 1978, *9,* 77–84.

Caccamo, J. M. Speech, language, and audiological services—An inalienable right. *Language, Speech, and Hearing Services in Schools,* 1974, *5,* 173–175.

Dublinske, S. PL 94-142 due process decisions. *Asha,* 1980, *22,* 335–338.

Dublinske, S., & Healey, W. C. PL 94-142: Questions and answers for the speech-language pathologist and audiologist. *Asha,* 1978, *20,* 188–205.

Gallup, G. The eleventh annual Gallup poll of the public's attitudes toward the public schools. *Phi Delta Kappan,* 1979, 39.

Gilhool, T. K. Education: An inalienable right. *Exceptional Children,* 1973, *39,* 597–609.

Hagerty, R., & Howard, T. *How to make federal mandatory special education work for you.* Springfield: Charles C Thomas, 1978.

Federal Advisory Service. *Handicapped requirements handbook.* Washington, D.C., 1979.

Healey, W. C. Notes from the associate secretary for school affairs. Buckley amend-ment sparks controversy: Parents and students gain access to school files. *Lan-guage, Speech, and Hearing Services in Schools,* 1975, *6,* 115–116.

Kuriloff, P., True, R., Kirp, D., & Buss, W. Legal reform and educational change: The Pennsylvania case. *Exceptional Children,* 1974, *41,* 35–42.

Melcher, J. W. Law, litigation, and handicapped children. *Exceptional Children,* 1976, *43,* 126–130.

Miller, S. Q., Miller, J. K., & Madison, C. L. A speech and language clinician's involvement in a PL 94-142 public hearing: A case study. *Language, Speech, and Hearing Services in Schools,* 1980, *11,* 75–84.

Pickering, M. The speech clinician and the family educational rights and privacy act of 1974. *Language, Speech, and Hearing Services in Schools,* 1976, *7,* 131–133.

Public Law 88-164, *Mental Retardation Facilities and Community Health Centers Construction Act of 1963.*

Public Law 89-10, *Elementary and Secondary Education Act of 1965.*

Public Law 89-750, *Elementary and Secondary Education Amendments of 1966.*

Public Law 91-230, *Education of the Handicapped Act of 1970.*

Public Law 93-112, *The Rehabilitation Act of 1973.*

Public Law 93-380, *Education Amendments of 1974.*

Public Law 94-142, *Education for All Handicapped Children Act of 1975.*

Reynolds, M. C. Staying out of jail. *Teaching Exceptional Children,* 1978, *10,* 60–62.

3

Identification and Assessment
of Communicatively Disordered Children

Before the actual class work is begun, there is still one more thing to be done. The teacher must meet each of the children who are to compose her speech classes and give to each a thorough examination. (Swift, 1972, p. 53)

This advice to speech correctionists initiating programs for the communicatively handicapped in the schools, recently reprinted, was first offered by Swift in the *Quarterly Journal of Speech Education* in 1919. The procedures advocated by Swift began with persuading school officials that a need existed for speech services; this was established through questionnaires sent to teachers in the district. The teachers were to indicate the names and addresses of all children thought to have speech disorders. According to Swift, this information was most convincing to educators. He said that three hundred children with speech disorders would probably be located in school systems employing one hundred teachers. Next, principals were asked to provide specific information about the students referred by the teachers. Then speech correctionists made comprehensive evaluations of each child and, if indicated, therapy was initiated. Participation in the therapeutic process by both teachers and parents was encouraged.

Although many years have intervened since Swift wrote about the beginning of speech correction programs in the schools, some similarities between procedures he advocated in 1919 and those still employed today are apparent. Seldom it is necessary for speech-language pathologists to convince administrators that communicatively disordered children exist. Although the precise incidence of communicative disorders among the various groups of children is unclear, such problems occur with frequency among the school age population. That services should be provided to these handicapped children must not be questioned. In order to qualify for federal assistance under PL 94-142, districts must meet the needs of these students. Swift suggested using questionnaires to locate communicatively impaired children; today, speech-language pathologists employ teacher referral, classroom visitation, and screening techniques to identify speech and language impaired individuals. Finally, Swift stated that a thorough evaluation must be completed before intervention was initiated; PL 94-142 requires that evaluative procedures confirm the presence and nature of communicative disorders.

Contemporary speech-language pathologists, then, have many of the same responsibilities as their 1919 counterparts did. They must identify and evaluate communicatively disordered children in the most efficient manner possible and plan and execute therapy based on their findings. This chapter considers identification and diagnostic procedures in an established speech-language therapy program. It is assumed that compliance with state and federal legislation makes it unnecessary to discuss the initiation of such programs. Following definitions of terms and consideration of anticipated incidences of speech, language, and hearing disorders, attention shifts to those techniques that may be employed in the identification and assessment of communicatively disordered children. Although certain procedural biases may be detected by the reader, no conscious attempt is made to advocate one technique over another.

DEFINITIONS

When considering the various communicative disorders, speech-language pathologists classify clients according to the presenting deviant communicative behaviors or according to the etiology of such behaviors. An individual with an articulatory disorder has difficulty in the production and use of speech sounds. Such a problem may be related to a single cause, or it may result from a combination of etiological factors. Although the cause of the problem will affect treatment options, it is critical that the overt behavior be accurately identified before etiology is considered. The professional who knows that a child has cerebral palsy may anticipate difficulty with language, phonation, hearing, rate of speech, and/or articulation. However, if that same child distorts /r/, is that deviation necessarily related to his or her neuromuscular condition? Or, if a child has a language disorder, is it the result of brain damage or could it be due to overprotectiveness of the part of the parents? In short, although etiology is significant in treatment, an accurate description of the specific communicative problems presented by the child is perhaps more informative. For the purposes of this text, a descriptive classification is employed.

Three terms require explanation; these are case finding, case selection, and case load. *Case finding* refers to the procedure whereby communicatively disordered children are identified. Evaluative procedures are then employed to confirm the presence of a specific problem and its severity. Traditionally, the techniques used to identify communicative disorders in children are screening, teacher referral, and classroom visitation. *Screening* involves a short conversation with each child in order to assess voice, fluency, language, and articulation in contextual speech; brief tests of language and/or articulation may also be administered. This procedure is intended to distinguish those children with possible communicative disorders from those whose communicative abilities are within the normal range. *Teacher referral* relies on the classroom teacher's identification of children with possible problems and subsequent referral of those students to the speech-language pathologist for evaluation. Finally, *classroom visitation* is sometimes employed as a means of case finding. Using this technique, the speech-language pathologist spends time in the classroom during periods of oral recitation. Children are identified as communicatively disordered on the basis of their performance in this natural setting. A more complete discussion of case finding appears later in this chapter.

Case selection, the second term which requires definition, refers to the process of determining which management alternative is preferable for each child presenting a communicative disorder. Finally, *case load* refers to the actual number of students being serviced directly by the speech-language pathologist. These two procedures are discussed in Chapter 4.

INCIDENCE DATA

Accurate information regarding the incidence of speech, language, and hearing disorders among school age children is not available despite the several attempts that have been made to collect such data. One early indication of the prevalence of speech, language, and hearing handicaps among children was reported by the Mid-Century White House Conference (American Speech and Hearing Association Committee on the Mid-Century White House Conference, 1952). As Table 3-1 shows, an incidence of 5 percent was obtained. It should be noted that only the most serious disorders were considered in this estimate; another 5 percent of the children between the ages of 5 and 21 were thought to have minor problems.

Milisen (1971) reported that the estimated incidence of speech defects among children ranged from 1.0 percent (in Philadelphia) to 21.4 percent (in Fresno, California). Other estimates of the prevalence of communicative

Table 3-1
Mid-Century White House Conference Estimate of
Communicative Disorders Among Children

Type of Disorder	Percentage of Children Presenting the Disorder
Articulatory	3.0
Fluency	.7
Vocal	.2
Cleft palate	.1
Cerebral palsy	.2
Linguistic	.3
Auditory with associated speech disorder	.5
Total Incidence	5.0

SOURCE: Adapted from American Speech and Hearing Association
Committee on the Mid-Century White House Conference, 1952.

disorders indicate that between 5 and 25 percent of all school age children
have significant speech disorders (Phillips, 1975). According to Phillips
(1975), "it is probably safe to judge that between 8 and 10 percent of the
children now enrolled in school exhibit some kind of oral communication
disorder" (p. 15).

When looking specifically at high school and college populations,
discrepancies become apparent. In 1939, a survey of Illinois high schools
revealed speech defects among 23.3 percent of the freshman, 21 percent of the
sophomores, 20 percent of the juniors, and 17.8 percent of the senior students
(Milisen, 1971). An earlier study indicated that only 1.3 percent of 224
freshmen had defective speech. In 1980, the speech-language abilities of 242
freshman students enrolled in a midwestern high school were assessed
(Southern Illinois University at Edwardsville, 1980). Of these students, 9 required complete evaluation, 10 presented temporary vocal deviations, and 7
had inconsistent misarticulations. Therefore, the incidence of significant
problems was 4 percent, with an additional 7 percent presenting minor differences. At the college level, estimates had varied from 3.9 percent to 18 percent (Milisen, 1971). Although multiple variables affect interpretation of incidence data, wide variation in reported estimates at all age levels is apparent.

As the preceding discussion suggests, little agreement is evident regarding the incidence of communicative disorders among school and college age
young people. A review of the incidence of specific communicative disorders
reveals similar discrepancies. Depending on the population assessed, the communicative behavior under scrutiny, the methods of assessment employed,
and the criteria for diagnosis, a variety of incidence figures is obtained.

According to Milisen (1971), for example, 15 to 20 percent of all first grade children present misarticulations. This incidence decreases as the age of the population surveyed increases; after the fourth grade, the number of children displaying articulatory problems appears to stabilize, with up to 3 percent of the students continuing to evidence such errors. Stuttering is assumed to affect about one percent of the school age population; studies of specific groups may reveal greater or lesser incidence figures, however. A 1976 survey by Brady and Hall suggests that the prevalence of stuttering is decreasing. These investigators found that only 0.35 percent of school children in K–12 displayed stuttering behavior; a higher incidence was found among retarded children. Vocal disorders present particular problems in incidence studies because of the sometimes subjective nature of assessment and temporary duration of the deviations. A conservative estimate is that one percent of the population is affected by vocal problems. Recent advances in evaluative methods in the area of language preclude the meaningful use of historical estimates of the incidence of linguistic disorders. The Mid-Century White House Conference, for example, suggested that less than one percent of all school age children present "retarded speech development." As the following discussion of case load distribution reveals, children with language disorders are being seen increasingly by speech-language pathologists. This does not necessarily imply that language disorders among children are on the increase but rather suggests that awareness of language disorders by speech-language pathologists is increasing. In summary, then, the results of surveys reporting the incidence of communicative disorders in general and the incidence of specific types of communicative disorders are difficult to analyze due to the numerous variables involved.

Another means of estimating the incidence of specific communicative disorders is through analysis of the composition of public school case loads. Black (1964) presented the distribution of disorders reported by clinicians in the state of Illinois during the 1962–1963 school year. At that time, 82 percent of the children enrolled for therapy presented disordered articulation. In descending order of occurrence were students displaying delayed speech (5 percent), vocal disorders (4 percent), stuttering (4 percent), hearing impairment (2 percent), and cleft palate, cerebral palsy, and aphasia (each one percent). No provision was made in the reporting procedures for the inclusion of children presenting multiple disorders.

A 1980 survey of public school speech-language pathologists indicated that the 61 reporting professionals were responsible for approximately 56,779 children (Hahn, 1980). Of that population, 6 percent had been identified as having communicative disorders and were involved in either direct intervention or alternative management programs for those problems. The distribution of specific disorders within the case load is presented in Table 3-2.

Comparing this case load distribution to that reported by Black, the

Table 3-2
Case Load Distribution of 61 Reporting
School Speech-Language Pathologists

Type of Disorder	Percentage of Children in Case Load Presenting the Disorder
Articulatory	50
Language	39
Auditory	4
Fluency	4
Voice	3

SOURCE: Data from Hahn, 1980.

most significant variation is seen in the incidence of language disorders. The first survey indicated that only 5 percent of the children seen in the early 1960s presented language problems; the 1980 survey showed that 39 percent of the case load displayed such disorders. A decrease in articulatory disorders is seen from 1962 to 1980, while distribution of other disorders remains somewhat constant. When these similarities and differences in case load distribution are analyzed, the increase in language disorders is not surprising. The school speech-language pathologist of the 1960s was ill-equipped to deal with children presenting such problems. Moreover, training programs were just beginning to emphasize language as a part of the curriculum. The decrease in the number of children being seen for articulatory disorders does not necessarily suggest that such problems are occurring with less frequency. Rather, this may reflect a modification of intervention emphasis on the part of practicing speech-language pathologists.

Speech-language pathologists in the schools, then, continue to function in ways reminiscent of their 1919 counterparts. Although the types of problems being handled are somewhat different, it remains the speech-language pathologist's responsibility to identify and assess all children presenting deviations in communicative ability.

CASE FINDING

Single Person Screening

There are a variety of ways to identify children with communicative disorders. One method is the screening, or survey, technique. Using this procedure, the speech-language pathologist sees each child individually in an effort to determine if the child's communicative abilities are within the normal range. Prior to the survey, specific arrangements are necessary. Initially, some determination of the population to be screened is required. Usually, this population includes transfers to the school, children who have received services in the preceding year, teacher referrals, and students at predetermined grade levels. The grades to be screened may be determined by district or state regulations, program supervisors, or the individual speech-language pathologist. Although it is typical to survey first graders, children at other levels (including kindergarten) may be involved. Next, the speech-language pathologist must arrange for suitable physical accommodations. It is desirable for the children to be seen in the "speech room," but the location of that room in the building may preclude such a luxury. More than one first grader has been temporarily lost in his or her attempt to find a speech room located on a different floor or in another section of the building. Alternatives to seeing children in the speech room include working in the classroom itself (a highly distracting option), finding a vacant room close to the classroom to be surveyed, or "setting up shop" in the hallway outside of the classroom. Working in a nearby vacant room is clearly the most attractive option.

Insofar as the sequence of screening is concerned, the following procedures are logical. Those children who received services in the preceding year may be screened first. Although these students will have IEPs, responsible speech-language pathologists may want to assess their status after the summer vacation. These students can usually be located easily and are not threatened by being removed from the classroom. Transfers to the school should be seen next; they are frequently older children who may not be anxious about the experience. Classroom surveys can then be conducted. Postponing the screening allows the children to become more comfortable in the school setting; this may be particularly important when the screenings are to take place at the kindergarten level. Finally, the children referred by teachers should be seen.

Additional preparations are necessary for classrom surveys. Initially, the speech-language pathologist arranges with the classroom teacher for a convenient time for the screening and obtains a list of the students' names. Arrangements may be made for each child to wear a name tag. Frequently, it is difficult to understand children when they say their names; some children may not know both their first and last names. The screening may proceed in alphabetical order. The speech-language pathologist obtains a list from the teacher and begins with the first child. Upon completion of each screening, the child is told whom to send out next. Having screening notes in alphabetical order can save time in completing reports.

Having made preliminary decisions regarding the logistics of case finding procedures, the speech-language pathologist must determine which materials and methods will be employed during the survey. To be effective, the procedures should provide a sufficient speech and language sample to assess articulation in single words and conversation and to allow for analysis of each child's linguistic competence and vocal and rhythmic attributes. In addition, the speech-language pathologist should be able to make a clinical judgment relative to the child's hearing acuity. Moreover, the procedure should be brief but sufficiently sensitive to determine whether the child's communicative abilities are within the acceptable range.

Materials and procedures that may be employed during the screening are varied. Commercial tools may be used as well as clinician-prepared materials. Several instruments may be employed for assessing articulation. The Bryngelson-Glaspey test, although not one of the more recently developed instruments, is an example of a screening test of articulation. It is designed to assess the child's production of the more commonly misarticulated phonemes. A brief test, the Bryngelson-Glaspey provides a quick assessment of the child's ability to produce 16 frequently used phonemes in single words. Other tests considered to be diagnostic in nature have screening sections. The Templin-Darley Diagnostic Tests of Articulation, for example, include a screening portion; the length of this test portion, however, precludes its use in the school setting, where brevity is important. The Fisher-Logemann Test of Articulation Competence also has a screening section. One instrument, the Predictive Screening Test of Articulation, has been found to be prognostic in distinguishing which children will overcome their articulatory errors without intervention from those whose misarticulations will persist (Van Riper & Erickson, 1969). Many speech-language pathologist opt not to use a commercial test but instead rely on materials they have prepared. Others have found that asking the child to count, identify colors and shapes, and/or tell about a favorite TV show provides satisfactory results. It should be emphasized that any screening procedure must include a contextual sample of speech production; single-word responses to objects or pictures do not provide adequate samples for analysis of articulatory competence.

In assessing language competence, screening tools are also available. Hutchinson, Hanson, and Mecham (1979) identify the following as screening tests: Bankson Screening Test, Northwestern Syntax Screening Test, Reynell Developmental Language Scales, Structured Photographic Language Test, the Utah Test of Language Development. Unfortunately for the school speech-language pathologist, these tests require from 15 to 30 minutes to administer and may not be appropriate for the identification process. Therefore, many speech-language pathologists base their clinical judgments of language competence on the language sample obtained during the screening. Others may devise their own screening tests. Again, because this is an identifying procedure, those students presenting language differences or deviations must be seen for a thorough evaluation, at which time formal tests are administered; parental consent is needed for this assessment.

In the areas of voice and rhythm, the speech-language pathologist also relies on clinical judgments. Vocal disorders may be temporary, and the speech-language pathologist should assess children with such problems on more than one occasion. Similarly, a follow-up assessment of children presenting dysfluent speech should be made. Students with suspected auditory impairments should be seen for audio-metric evaluation and/or referred for further testing.

The foregoing discussion relates to screening done by the speech-language pathologist who is assigned to one or more schools. All children at specific grade levels, children new to the school, children previously enrolled in therapy, children on the underserved list, and children referred by teachers are seen by the speech-language pathologist for a preliminary assessment of their communicative abilities. Screening may also be accomplished by a team of professionals or by paraprofessionals.

Team Screenings

The *team screening* may take several forms. For example, a team screening may have multiple purposes; it may involve not only screening for speech and language defects but may include assessment of other skills such as reading readiness or motoric abilities. Such screenings are typically conducted at the preschool level by professionals representing a variety of disciplines. These professionals are located at stations within a facility and the children move from station to station. Children failing to display normal functioning in one or more areas may be evaluated at that time or scheduled for complete evaluation at a later date. The screening procedures utilized by the speech-language pathologist in a group screening would essentially be the same as for single person screenings. The materials employed would be consistent with the characteristics of the population, and the decision to conduct further evaluations would be based on the adequacy of the child's communicative abilities.

Another type of team screening is that carried out for a single purpose by two or more speech-language pathologists. These professionals might be assigned to screen a particular group of children specified by grade level or might survey an entire school. For example, a group of five speech-language pathologists might enter a school containing six first-grade classrooms; the purpose of the screening would be the location of children with suspected communicative disorders. With this type of screening, several factors in addition to those already discussed must be considered. Critical to the success of team screening is agreement among the participants on procedures and criteria for failure. Individuals involved in the testing must determine whether formal tests will be used and, if so, which instruments. Of even greater importance is agreement as to what constitutes a communicative disorder. Although this issue is addressed in greater detail in a later chapter, it is important at this point to consider the fact that professionals do differ in their concepts of communicative disorders even at the identification stage. In a group speech and language screening, then, it is important to establish some criteria for making consistent judgments. For example, the professionals involved might determine that a five-year-old child must misarticulate two phonemes below his developmental level in at least two positions to be considered as having an articulatory problem. Consensus as to developmental norms would be required when such a criterion is established.

Similar consensus is necessary in the area of language. The population to be assessed might dictate the criteria established for determining language competency. For example, should the same criteria be applied to inner city children, suburban children, and children residing in rural areas? This question is without a conclusive answer, but certainly it should be asked when criteria for judging a specific population are under consideration. Vocal conditions present particular problems in team screenings. Subjective judgments frequently determine the adequacy and appropriateness of voice. Professionals sometimes vary in the amount of deviation they accept. For the most part, speech-language pathologists would agree in their judgments of children with gross deviations; however, less obvious problems in the areas of phonation, resonance, and intensity might not always be of concern to professionals involved in a team screening. Because consistency in the identification of communicatively disordered children is desirable, the criteria for making such judgments should be established in advance.

A 1973 report on rapid screening procedures describes in detail the execution of three types of screenings (American Speech and Hearing Association, 1973). The first, the classroom survey, has already been discussed. Small-group screening is recommended for use with special populations including preschoolers and children enrolled in special education classes. With this technique, the students are seen in small groups of from three to eight children, rather than individually. Each child is asked to tell his name, identify certain body parts, and name and describe pictures. The task force suggests utilization of this technique when other rapid screening procedures may be ineffective. The final method involves team screening using supportive personnel. Either properly trained volunteers or paid paraprofessionals may participate. The children are assessed using predetermined and uniform procedures and are evaluated on a pass-fail basis; those children failing the screening are referred for a thorough evaluation.

It is apparent, then, that not all team screenings are conducted by certified speech-language pathologists. A perusal of the literature reveals that paraprofessionals are sometimes employed to facilitate the process; the credentials of these individuals differ, and the question of the amount and type of training required to prepare such people continues to be debated. Nevertheless, reports describing the functioning of supportive personnel are available and should be considered by the speech-language pathologist.

Dopheide and Dallinger (1976) described the utilization of parents in screening their prekindergarten children for articulatory errors. In advance of a kindergarten registration program, parents were sent a copy of the Denver Articulation Screening Exam (DASE), with instructions for administering and scoring the test. They were instructed to administer the exam to their children and return the results on the day of the registration. Complete results were obtained on 73 of the 87 preregistered children. As a part of the multiple-purpose screening, the DASE was readministered to each child by a trained aide or the speech-language pathologist. The test administrators were not aware of the results reported by the parents. In comparing the results of the parent-administered test with those of the aide–clinician, substantial agreement was found. Of the 46 parents reporting that their children made no articulatory errors on the DASE, 82 percent were accurate when compared with the clinician-aide assessments. Of those parents reporting errors on the DASE, similar accuracy was not reported. Nevertheless, the researchers were guardedly optimistic about the role that parents might play in the assessment of their children's articulatory skills.

Pickering and Dopheide (1976) reported on the training of school personnel to conduct speech and language screening in rural areas of Maine. Two-day workshops were held twice to train 37 aides; none of the school personnel had any background in speech and language. The competency based workshops were conducted by CCC-SP instructors. The objectives of the workshops, presented behaviorally, related to the participants' abilities to score the Templin-Darley Screening Test of Articulation and to identify communicative disorders from recorded speech samples. Participants were also afforded opportunities to demonstrate achievement of these objectives under the supervision of a speech-language pathologist. In evaluating the training program after the personnel had participated in actual screenings, it was apparent that the trainees tended to overrefer children. The reason for that tendency was unclear. Additional information regarding the use of school personnel in speech and language screenings is needed, but the results of this training program are encouraging.

With the awareness that supportive personnel are now participating in therapy programs, the question arises as to whether they should be allowed to identify children with speech and language problems. Van Riper's (1969) classic definition of a speech (language) disorder states that "Speech is defective when it deviates so far from the speech of other people that it calls attention to itself, interferes with communication, or causes its possessor to be maladjusted" (p. 29). If one accepts this description of disordered communication, then justification for using supportive personnel in the identification process can be found. If the lay person or trained paraprofessional cannot identify an individual with a communicative disorder, does a handicapping condition actually exist? "Deviant speech is a problem not because it is different, but because it impairs emotional, social, or economic well-being.

When it does not, it is merely different, not handicapping" (Clase, 1976, p. 51). The question here is whether there are occasions when speech-language pathologists identify problems which are not obvious to or even identifiable by lay persons. In the area of articulation, an eight-year-old boy with a distorted /r/ may be used as an example. Speech-language pathologists would be very aware of such a problem, but would the lay person be equally aware and concerned about that deviation? If the answer to that question is "no," then are speech-language pathologists creating problems? If the child's communicative abilities are not diminished by the /r/ distortion, if he is intelligible to others, if he is not troubled by the problem, then is there any need for intervention? Is the problem, then, a problem? Regarding fluency, it has been noted that the initial diagnosis of stuttering is frequently made by a lay person. Therefore, paraprofessionals would certainly identify stuttering children; in fact, they might overidentify children who are dysfluent. Many speech-language pathologists feel uncomfortable in diagnosing vocal disorders. Lay persons might also be somewhat weak in this area. With regard to language, it cannot be assumed that paraprofessionals will recognize all differences in language structure. These individuals may be accurate in identifying significant deviations but may miss some of the more subtle differences. It would appear, therefore, that uniform testing procedures would be appropriate if paraprofessionals were to be employed in screening for language disorders.

The survey or screening method of case finding, then, may be conducted in a variety of ways. A single speech-language pathologist or a group of professionals may be involved. Recent literature describes the utilization of supportive personnel in the screening process. There are some obvious problems involved in using lay persons, but speech-language pathologists should not dismiss this possibility. Similar problems are inherent in the next method discussed, teacher referral, which also requires the participation of lay persons.

Teacher Referral

A popular technique for case finding is that of *teacher referral*. It is more frequently used at the higher grade levels than the screening procedures already described. When using the teacher referral method, teachers should receive inservice training, ideally through a series of sessions conducted by the school speech-language pathologist. These meetings are designed to familiarize the teachers with the nature and characteristics of communicative disorders. This could be part of a total inservice program which would not only consider identification of children with speech and language deviations but would also describe the classroom teachers' roles in intervention. The information given to the teachers should include material on the various disorders and examples of each. The teachers can then be asked to refer to the speech-language pathologist any children in their classrooms who may present speech, language, or hearing problems. Normally, the teacher referral method requires more time, since it may be several weeks into the school year before the teachers have had sufficient opportunity to listen to the children and to make judgments regarding their communicative skills.

Several studies have been conducted to test the efficiency of the teacher referral method. Nodar (1978) evaluated the abilities of the classroom teachers of 2231 school age children to identify hearing impairments in those students. Using observation of classroom behavior as a criterion, the teachers were able to identify some children with hearing losses who had not been detected by pure tone audiometry. Contrary to the findings of earlier studies, which reported that teachers are not sensitive to auditory disorders, Nodar found teachers to be valuable in identifying hearing impaired children and recommended that they be included on the screening team.

Stilling (1972) studied 30 elementary and middle school teachers' abilities to identify articulatory disorders from audiotaped samples. None of the teachers had had any coursework in speech and language pathology but, prior to listening to the tapes, they had read material describing articulatory errors. Two speech-language pathologists also evaluated the tapes. Agreement between the teachers and the speech-language pathologists of 75 percent was achieved. This percentage was no greater than that reported in earlier studies in which no preliminary information had been given to the teachers. Nevertheless, the researcher suggested that "speech clinicians should consider that not only might teachers overlook speech handicapped children, but the clinicians might have lost perspective in what constitutes a speech problem" (Stilling, 1972, p. 28).

In a similar study, 50 classroom teachers were asked to identify children with defective speech from tape recordings of 10 students (Clausen & Kopatic, 1975). Four children presented normal communication and six exhibited disorders of fluency, voice, language, and articulation. The results showed that 28 percent of the teachers failed to identify the normal speech of one of the 10 subjects; further, 82 percent did not detect the dysfluency of a 10-year-old stuttering child. The overall accuracy of the teachers in identifying normal and defective speech was approximately 72 percent.

Finally, Wertz and Mead (1975) compared the severity ratings of speech disorders assigned by classroom teachers and speech-language pathologists. The severity of 20 15-second taperecorded samples of children with vocal disorders, cleft palate speech, articulatory problems, or fluency disturbances was rated by 96 teachers and 24 speech-language pathologists. Both classroom teachers and speech-language pathologists rated stuttering as the most serious disorder, with vocal disturbances being considered the least severe. Interestingly, as a group, the teachers displayed more agreement among themselves than did the speech-language pathologists.

Teacher referral, then, is a case finding technique that relies on the classroom teacher to identify and refer children with suspected communicative disorders. Its efficiency rate appears to be at about the 75 percent level. Although it would be assumed that the 75 percent would include all children with serious problems, this may not always be true. It would appear, therefore, that this technique should supplement the survey method rather than serve as the single procedure for case finding.

Classroom Visitation

The final method of case finding cited in the literature is *classroom visitation*. Using this technique, the speech-language pathologist visits the classroom during periods of oral recitation and makes judgments relative to the adequacy of each child's communicative ability. Sometimes, oral reading serves as the sample to be analyzed. Since reading is not always reflective of conversational speech, this technique is ineffective. Any of you reading this passage now, if asked to read aloud, would present a very different communicative pattern as you read than you would during conversation. The stilted nature of reading, then, would not lend itself to sampling the child's communicative abilities. Additional problems might be encountered in having the opportunity to hear each child talk and in identifying each speaker. Although classroom visitation might be an effective technique in evaluating the carryover of a child's newly learned communicative skill, it does not appear to be an efficient case finding technique.

Preferred Case Finding Techniques

Having examined the identification options available to the speech-language pathologist, we need some indication of the relative popularity of these techniques. In an early study, Roe, Hanley, Crotty, and Mayper (1961) reported that the survey and teacher referral methods were employed most frequently. Regional differences were found in the 705 speech-language pathologists' responses to these investigators' survey. The screening method was utilized most frequently in the midwest, whereas west coast speech-language pathologists employed teacher referral extensively. The 141 supervisors responding to a similar survey acknowledged preference for the survey and teacher referral methods also.

A 1980 survey of 61 public school speech-language pathologists yielded interesting results (Hahn, 1980). A questionnaire was devised to determine whether case finding techniques differed at the various grade levels. At the preschool level, a combination of teacher referral and screening techniques was employed most frequently. Both teacher referral and a combination of teacher referral and screening were popular at the intermediate levels, with teacher referral dominating at the upper grade levels.

The efficiency of the various methods of case finding has been discussed throughout this section and requires no further consideration. It is important to note, however, that both regional differences and variations in grade levels appear to influence the preferred case finding techniques.

EVALUATION OF THE
COMMUNICATIVELY DISORDERED CHILD

Following the location of children with suspected communicative disorders, the speech-language pathologist must evaluate each child so identified. First, the parents should be informed that the child has been seen and that the results of the screening suggest that further testing is warranted. The parents must consent to an evaluation before it is initiated. In the event that permission is not granted, at least four alternatives are available; these options were discussed in Chapter 2. Once consent has been obtained, the speech-language pathologist must plan for the evaluation. PL 94-142 mandates that at least two methods must be utilized in making a diagnosis. This means, for example, that a child may not be diagnosed as having an articulatory disorder on the basis of a single test. The speech-language pathologist must administer a formal test of articulation and supplement that with an analysis of contextual speech. In addition, a case history must be prepared. Such a history may be obtained directly from an informant or prepared from materials made available to the speech-language pathologist. Although case history forms differ, it is customary to include educational background and medical and developmental history, as well as specific information related to the communicative problem. It is desirable if family and social histories can also be obtained. The reader is referred to Johnson, Darley, and Spriestersbach (1963), Hutchinson, Hanson, and Mecham (1979), and Sanders (1979) for examples of general and specific case history forms.

Following preparation of the case history, the speech-language pathologist must determine which diagnostic tools and techniques should be employed in the evaluation. Although the following discussion does not purport to be exhaustive, some indication of techniques appropriately utilized in the school setting appears necessary.

Assessment of Articulatory Skills

The initial identification of an articulatory disorder is usually made during conversation. A formal test of articulation should provide additional information about that defect. Numerous commercial tests are available. They differ in ease of administration and scoring, format, and administrative time required, as well as in test philosophy. Such tests may be designed to analyze articulation in terms of distinctive features (Fisher-Logemann Test of Articulation Competence) or developmental norms (Templin-Darley Diagnostic Tests of Articulation); to assess according to the frequency of occurrence of various phonemes in American English (The Arizona Articulation Proficiency Scale); to obtain multiple responses (Goldman-Fristoe Test of Articulation); or to analyze articulatory skills in terms of phonological processing (The Assessment of Phonological Processes).

Ease of administration, time required to administer the test, and ease of scoring were mentioned as criteria for test selection. The first factor might be individually determined; certainly practice in using a specific tool would improve efficiency in administration. Little research has compared the time required to administer the various tests. One study, however, compared the time required to administer the Goldman-Fristoe Test of Articulation and the Arizona Articulation Proficiency Scale (Whitehead & Mullen, 1975). Although the latter test contains 13 more stimulus plates than the former, the Arizona scale was more rapidly administered to 9 of the 10 subjects involved. The researcher attributed this finding to ambiguity of some of the stimulus pictures on the Goldman-Fristoe; even though this test has fewer plates, the time for administering it was greater.

With regard to ease of scoring, preferences may again be related to experience with the tool. The Goldman-Fristoe, for example, is considered by many to be difficult to score. Similar observations have been made by those using phonological process analysis. However, once the examiner becomes familiar with the system, scoring is facilitated. Moreover, if the information gained from analysis of the data is meaningful and will be of use in preparing the IEP, then it is certainly well worth the complications of the scoring method.

It has been assumed that all tests of articulation measure what they purport to test. Schissel and James (1979) conducted a study that makes this assumption questionable. Comparing the responses of 29 children to both the Arizona scale and the McDonald Deep Test of Articulation, the researchers found the former to be less sensitive. The results indicated that the Arizona scale failed to detect some children who made consistent articulatory errors on relatively few sounds. Therefore, the speech-language pathologist should be judicious in test selection with regard to the validity of the tool.

Many of the tests alluded to in the previous discussion involve picture-naming tasks. It was suggested that such tests should be supplemented by analysis of contextual speech. DuBois and Bernthal (1978) compared the efficiency of these two methods, as well as what they termed *modeled continuous speech*. The *continuous speech task* involved the child in telling a story about various stimulus pictures. The *modeled continuous speech task* required the child to include specific stimulus words in phrases or sentences. The *spontaneous picture-naming task* required the child to name stimulus pictures.

Not surprisingly, the researchers found that more errors were heard during the continuous speaking task; the fewest errors were elicited during picture naming. This finding should reaffirm the necessity for obtaining and analyzing a spontaneous speech sample.

Several attempts have been made to devise tests that are predictive in nature. Farquhar (1961) evaluated the imitative and auditory discrimination abilities of 50 kindergarten children with mild articulatory problems and 50 students with severe disorders. Seven months later, all children were reassessed; none had been involved in intervention during that period. The researcher reported that the ability to imitate was prognostically valuable with this group of children; results of the tests of auditory discrimination were not significant.

The Carter-Buck Tests of Stimulability, also designed to be prognostic, were the tools studied by Kisatsky (1967). The tests were administered to 82 kindergarten children who were then divided into high and low stimulability groups. After a six-month period without intervention, the two groups were reevaluated. The high stimulability groups demonstrated significant improvement over those children with low stimulability ratings. The predictive value of the tests, therefore, was confirmed.

Assessment of the articulatory skills of children, then, should include administration of a formal test of articulation, analysis of a contextual speech sample, and evaluation of stimulability. Audiometric testing is required, and supplementary tests of auditory discrimination and memory span may be administered. Finally, an assessment of the anatomy and physiology of the speech mechanism is indicated.

Assessment of Fluency

When the child presents a fluency disorder, a speech sample should be obtained and analyzed, but additional observations of the child's speech in different situations should also be made. The reader is well aware that stuttering varies significantly from stutterer to stutterer and fluctuates within the individual stutterer. The child may display severe dysfluencies in the classroom and be reasonably fluent at home; the reverse may also be true. It behooves the speech-language pathologist to obtain several samples of the child's speech prior to making a firm diagnosis.

In assessing the stuttering behavior, the nature of the dysfluencies should be noted. For example, the appearance and consistency of repetitions, prolongations, and/or interjections should be recorded. The speech-language pathologist should also attempt to identify any associated behaviors including tension, gaze aversion, and other secondary characteristics. The variations in stuttering in different situations should also be noted.

Checklists, self-inventories, and scales for rating the severity of stuttering are available to the speech-language pathologist. Among these are Riley's Stuttering Severity Instrument for Children and Adults, the Iowa Scale of Stuttering Severity, and Cooper's Chronicity Prediction Checklist. The reader is also referred to Johnson, Darley, and Spriestersbach (1963) for additional materials. Although a case history is an important part of any evaluation, its significance in assessing a young stutterer cannot be overemphasized. Therefore, a comprehensive evaluation should include direct and indirect observation of the child in a variety of situations, careful attention to the types of dysfluencies and related behaviors, and a meticulous case history. Only after all information has been analyzed can a diagnosis of stuttering be made.

Assessment of Voice

In the absence of sophisticated instrumentation, it is the ear of the speech-language pathologist that is critical in the assessment of children with possible vocal disorders. Judgments concerning the adequacy of a child's voice should be made on a number of occasions. The child who is hoarse, for example, may be susceptible to allergies. A child may have a cold at the time of the initial screening and may not present a chronic vocal disorder. Therefore, the speech-language pathologist must make several observations before proceeding.

Several checklists are available for evaluating vocal attributes. Some of these appear in Johnson et al. (1963). A comprehensive description of diagnostic procedures involving both instrumental and subjective assessments may be found in Hutchinson, Hanson, and Mecham (1979). The latter authors discuss specific procedures for identifying problems associated with respiratory differences, as well as techniques for analyzing pitch, intonation, loudness, and quality. They note that "we can supply guidelines and specific procedures but recognition of the occurrence of harmful pitch, tensions, or defects of loudness or qualities cannot be developed by reading a book" (Hutchinson et al., 1979, p. 227).

The case history is again important in the evaluation of a child with a suspected vocal disorder. Since medical clearance must be sought in cases in which a pathology may be present, early referral is imperative. It is the responsibility of the speech-language pathologist to identify such problems and to obtain a confirming diagnosis from an otolaryngologist prior to initiating therapy.

Assessment of Hearing

The identification of children with hearing impairment may or may not be the responsibility of the school speech-language pathologist, depending upon the regulations of the school district. In some systems, hearing screenings are conducted by public health officials or the school nurse. Those children identified as hearing impaired are referred to an audiologist for complete evaluation. Speech-language pathologists may be responsible for testing the hearing of children in their case loads. Since these individuals usually do not have the instrumentation needed to perform sophisticated assessments, it is necessary to refer children failing the screening to certified audiologists.

Assessment of Language

In the area of language, the case history assumes tremendous importance. Accuracy in obtaining information from the parent or guardian is essential to a diagnosis. Informant interviews may be utilized to supplement information contained in the case history. The Verbal Language Development Scale may be used when the communicative abilities of children up to 15 years are under consideration. Informal testing, such as that employed during the screening, may be expanded. Objects and pictures can serve as the stimuli, with the child's utterances being recorded and analyzed. There are a variety of ways to obtain and analyze language samples depending on the information desired. Barrie-Blackley, Musselwhite, and Rogister (1978) discuss issues in language sampling and describe a protocol for transcription and analysis. Sanders (1979) also presents a lucid discussion of language sampling techniques.

In addition to informant interviews, informal testing, and language sampling techniques, the speech-language pathologist may use numerous tests to evaluate general and specific abilities. Tests such as the Test of Language Development, The Houston Test of Language Development, and the Utah Test of Language Development purport to assess a variety of linguistic abilities. Receptive vocabulary may be assessed using the Peabody Picture Vocabulary Test or the Quick Test. Among the tests measuring syntactic skills are the Northwestern Syntax Screening Test and the Carrow Elicited Language Inventory. Bloom and Lahey (1978) discuss methods of assessing pragmatic skills in their book.

In evaluating the child with a language problem, then, the speech-language pathologist has access to an increasing number of tools and techniques. The tests mentioned in the previous discussion may be appropriately utilized in the school setting, but there are others of equal value. The purpose of the assessment, the age of the child, and the nature of the problem should be considered in test selection.

Referrals

An important part of the diagnostic process is determining which children should be referred for additional evaluation. The Code of Ethics of the American Speech-Language-Hearing Association prevents speech-language pathologists from becoming involved in areas in which they are not sufficiently trained. Although overreferral may become a problem, it is preferable to err on the side of overreferring children with possible medical or emotional problems than to underrefer. As pointed out earlier, children with vocal problems involving a suspected pathology must be referred for evaluation by an otolaryngologist. The child with a hearing impairment should be seen by an audiologist and an otologist. The child with a language disorder may or may not be referred to a psychometrist or psychologist; the same is true of a child who presents a fluency disturbance.

Most school districts now have teams of professional personnel who can perform a variety of evaluations. Some children seen by the speech-language pathologist may require assessment by such a team. Frequently this evaluation is followed by development of a prescriptive intervention program and trial placement in a classroom that provides the services felt to be necessary.

It is important that the speech-language pathologist be cognizant of the various resources available for placement of a child not only within the school district, but within the community as well. There will be occasions when the services provided by the speech-language pathologist will not be commensurate with the needs of the child. The needs of a severely language-delayed child, for example, might not be met by the itinerant speech-language pathologist. In such a case, placement in a special language classroom would be preferable. It is also possible that the needs of that child might best be met in a facility outside of the school district. The speech-language pathologist must keep these sources of referral in mind when making decisions about children diagnosed as communicatively disordered.

REFERENCES

American Speech and Hearing Association Committee on the Mid-Century White House Conference. Speech disorders and speech correction. *Journal of Speech and Hearing Disorders,* 1952, *17,* 129–137.

American Speech and Hearing Association. Task force report on school speech, hearing, and language screening procedures. *Language, Speech, and Hearing Services in Schools,* 1973, *4,* 109–119.

Barrie-Blackley, S., Musselwhite, C. R., & Rogister, S. *Clinical language sampling.* Danville: The Interstate Printers and Publishers, Inc. 1978.

Black, M. *Speech correction in the schools.* Englewood Cliffs: Prentice-Hall, 1964.

Bloom, L., & Lahey, M. *Language development and language disorders.* New York: John Wiley, 1978.

Brady, W., & Hall, D. The prevalence of stuttering among school-age children. *Language, Speech, and Hearing Services in Schools,* 1976, *7,* 75–81.

Clase, J. Ethical implications of screening. *Language, speech and hearing services in schools,* 1976, *7,* 50–55.

Clauson, G., & Kopatic, N. Teacher attitudes and knowledge of remedial speech programs. *Language, Speech and Hearing Services in Schools.* 1975, *6,* 206–211.

Dopheide, W. R., & Dallinger, J. R. Preschool articulation screening by parents.
Language, Speech, and Hearing Services in Schools. 1976, *7,* 124–127.

DuBois, E. M., & Bernthal, J. E. A comparison of three methods for obtaining articulatory responses. *Journal of Speech and Hearing Disorders,* 1978, *43,* 295–305.

Farquhar, M. S. Prognostic value of imitative and auditory discrimination tests.
Journal of Speech and Hearing Disorders. 1961, *26,* 342–347.

Hahn, C. An investigation into current procedures of case finding, case selection and
scheduling in the schools. Unpublished M.S. thesis, Southern Illinois University at
Edwardsville, 1980.

Hutchinson, B., Hanson, M. L., & Mecham, M. J. *Diagnostic handbook of speech
pathology.* Baltimore: The Williams and Wilkins Company, 1979.

Johnson, W., Darley, F. L., & Spriestersbach, D. C. *Diagnostic methods in speech
pathology.* New York: Harper & Row, Publishers, 1963.

Kisatsky, T. J. The prognostic value of Carter-Buck tests in measuring articulation
skills of selected kindergarten children. *Exceptional Children,* 1967, *34,* 81–85.

Milisen, R. The incidence of speech disorders. In L. E. Travis (Ed.), *Handbook of
speech pathology and audiology.* New York: Appleton-Century-Crofts, 1971.

Nodar, R. H. Teacher identification of elementary school children with hearing loss.
Language, Speech, and Hearing Services in Schools, 1978, *9,* 24–28.

Phillips, P. P. *Speech and hearing problems in the classroom.* Lincoln: Cliff Notes,
Inc., 1975.

Pickering, M., & Dopheide, W. R. Training aides to screen children for speech and
language problems. *Language, Speech, and Hearing Services in Schools,* 1976, *7,*
236–241.

Roe, V., Hanley, C. N., Crotty, C., & Mayper, L. Clinical practice: Diagnosis and
measurement. *Journal of Speech and Hearing Disorders Monograph Supplement*
8, 1961, 50–57.

Sanders, L. J. *Procedure Guides for Evaluation of Speech and Language Disorders in
Children* (4th ed.). Danville: The Interstate Printers and Publishers, Inc., 1979.

Schissel, R. J., & James, L. B. A comparison of children's performance on two tests of
articulation. *Journal of Speech and Hearing Disorders,* 1979, *44,* 363–372.

Southern Illinois University at Edwardsville. *Case Records,* 1980.

Stilling, C. M. A study of the agreement of classroom teachers with speech clinicians in
identifying children who have errors of articulation. *The Illinois Speech and Hearing Association Journal,* 1972, *6,* 25–28.

Swift, W. B. How to begin speech correction in the public schools. *Quarterly Journal
of Speech Education,* 1919. Reprinted in *Language, Speech, and Hearing Services
in Schools,* 1972, *3,* 51–56.

Van Riper, C. *Speech Correction Principles and Methods* (5th ed.). Englewood Cliffs:
Prentice-Hall, Inc., 1972.

Van Riper C., & Erickson, R. A predictive screening test of articulation. *Journal of
Speech and Hearing Disorders,* 1969, *34,* 214–219.

Wertz, R. T., & Mead M. D. Classroom teacher and speech clinician severity ratings of
different speech disorders. *Language, Speech, and Hearing Services in Schools,*
1975, *6,* 119–124.

Whitehead, R. L., & Mullen, P. A. A comparison of the administration times of two tests of articulation. *Language, Speech, and Hearing Services in Schools,* 1975, *6,* 150–153.

4

Case Selection
and Management Alternatives

The most competent speech clinician in the schools cannot be considered effective if he is working with the wrong children. Said differently, all the best techniques and skills in the world are of no consequence if wasted on those not needing it and denied to those who do. (Sommers, 1969, p. 250)

Prior to the implementation of PL 94-142, speech-language pathologists in the schools screened the target population using techniques described in the preceding chapter and then, using district, state, or personal guidelines, selected a predetermined number of students for inclusion in the active case load. Decisions to include some children and eliminate others may have been based on the speech-language pathologist's skill (or lack thereof) in managing specific kinds of disorders, the vehemence with which teachers and parents sought services for communicatively disordered children, the severity of the various problems, the age of a child, the number of children presenting problems, the teacher's willingness to release children from the classroom, or variations or combinations of these factors. Those children who were not selected for direct intervention were conveniently placed on a "waiting list." Some matured sufficiently while on this list to be dismissed; others were assimilated into the active case load when vacancies occurred. Today districts that have waiting lists are not in compliance with PL 94-142. Nevertheless, many speech-language pathologists are still responsible for more children than they can legally or ethically provide with appropriate service. Some alternative management plans are, therefore, necessary.

CASE LOAD

When the author was a school speech-language pathologist in the early 1960s, the state of Illinois had established 100 students as the maximum case load, 70 as the minimum. The method by which these numbers were selected was unknown, and justification for establishing such limitations would be difficult. Consider, for example, the speech-language pathologist working with multiply handicapped children; could that person achieve effective results seeing 70 severely involved children each week? Assuming that the average school day does not exceed six hours, the speech-language pathologist could conduct 12 half-hour sessions or 18 20-minute sessions each day. It is obvious that the needs of these 70 students could not be met. And the speech-language pathologist assigned to several rural schools might have additional difficulty maintaining an active case load of 70 students because of the time lost in traveling between schools. Therefore, the establishment of specific maximum and minimum case load figures seems inappropriate. It would appear that individual decisions based on the types and severity of the communicative disorders, the ages of the children presenting the problems, and the number of schools assigned would be a more justifiable means of determining the case load. Nevertheless, case load size continues often to be mandated and must be a consideration for the speech-language pathologist.

It is a positive trend that case loads appear to be decreasing. A survey of over 1400 public school speech-language pathologists in the late 1950s revealed that the mean case load was approximately 130 children (Bingham, Van Hattum, Faulk, and Toussig, 1961). At that time, west coast and northeastern speech-language pathologists reported the highest case loads, with the Southwest-Mountain States-Hawaii region and the Midwest reporting fewer students. That same survey revealed that 25 percent of the speech-language pathologists had their case loads limited by state law; an additional 5 percent reported local restrictions. Of those responding to the survey, 23 percent reported that the number of children requiring services determined the case load; apparently no minimum or maximum figures were utilized. Finally, 45 percent of the speech-language pathologists employed professional judgment in establishing case loads.

Among the changes O'Toole and Zaslow (1969) noted in describing the changing roles of the speech-language pathologist was a substantial reduction in case load size. In a school district, the following case loads were identified: one speech-language pathologist worked with 37 children, many of whom were cerebral palsied; a second speech-language pathologist had a case load of 45; and each of three speech-language pathologists worked with 10 or fewer hearing impaired children. These figures are in contrast to the mean case loads reported in the 1959 survey by Bingham et al. (1961).

Hoopes and Dasovich (1972) surveyed 76 public school speech-language pathologists. The majority, 47, were employed in a county school district; 29 worked in the city school district. Although the survey was a multipurpose one, one of the 17 pieces of information obtained revealed differences between the speech-language pathologists employed by the city and those working in the county; that item dealt with case load size. It was found that 52 percent of the city speech-language pathologists carried case loads of 100, but none of the county speech-language pathologists had case loads that high. Of the county speech-language pathologists, 57 percent reported case loads between 51 and 80. Only 7 percent of the city speech-language pathologists had comparable loads. Of both groups, 38 percent carried case loads between 81 and 99. In a 1976 study, the average case load of the reporting speech-language pathologists was aproximately 72 (Neal, 1976).

Hahn (1980) surveyed 61 speech-language pathologists nationwide. Only one of the 48 professionals responding to the question on case load reported carrying a case load above 90 students. Additional results are shown in Table 4-1.

Contemporary school speech-language pathologists seem to be servicing fewer students than did the professional of the late 1950s. In part, this reduction in case load may be the result of state recognition that effective therapy requires some degree of intensity. The state of Illinois, for example, now has no minimum for case loads and has established 80 as the maximum. North Dakota recommends a case load between 50 and 60, and fewer students are seen "if the communication disorders of the population being served warrants it" (North Dakota Department of Public Instruction, 1977, p. 5). Missouri specifies that the itinerant speech-language pathologist may service between 50 and 85 students (Missouri Special Education Services, 1977). Those speech-language pathologists assigned to resource rooms may see between 10 and 15 students; those working in self-contained rooms with children who have developmental speech and language disorders may see between 6 and 10 students. If a teacher aide is assigned, "it is possible that a broadened range of approved class size may be considered for the school district (Missouri Special Education Services, 1977, p. 14). PL 94-142 has also contributed to case load reduction.

The American Speech-Language-Hearing Association has attempted to provide guidelines for the establishment of uniform case load size or staff–pupil ratio. The American Speech and Hearing Association (1973–1974) has described nine variables that should be considered when determining case load size. These include (1) the needs of each communicatively disordered child; (2) the availability of programs and scheduling models; (3) the total responsibilities of the speech-language pathologist; (4) the number of students needing assistance; (5) the geographic area being serviced; (6) the socio-economic nature of the community; (7) the availability of paraprofessionals; (8) the number of special educators available; and (9) the support given the

Table 4-1
Case Loads Reported by 48
Speech-Language Pathologists

Case Load Size	No. of Speech-Language Pathologists
Fewer than 45 students	25
45 to 65 students	17
66 to 90 students	5
90 students or more	1
Total	48

SOURCE: Data from Hahn, 1980.

program by administrators, supervisors, and clerical staff. Although these variables make it difficult to specify exact case load recommendations, several suggestions are presented. In classrooms serving preschool deaf or language impaired children, the recommended teacher–pupil ratio is 1:6. Support services to hearing impaired children may be provided at a 1:12 ratio. The speech-language pathologist who serves cerebral palsied children may carry a case load of 25 students. Finally, the professional providing services to children presenting a variety of communicative disorders might be able to accommodate 50 to 60 students.

In summary, then, a variety of factors influence case load size. Those states specifying case load minima and maxima appear to be responding to the recommendations of local, state, and national professionals by reducing the maximum number. In some cases, minima are not specified. Ideally, the decision as to how many children can be serviced should be left to the discretion of the individual speech-language pathologist. Since this is not always the case, the school speech-language pathologist must be aware of case load regulations within the district and/or state, since case selection and assignment to the various management alternatives will be related to these restrictions.

CASE SELECTION

Case selection has always been a somewhat volatile issue among speech-language pathologists. Professionals have viewed the relative significance of the factors involved in this process from different perspectives. The type and severity of the disorder, the age of the child presenting the problem, and the social aspects of the deviations have all been considered. In this section, a review of the literature regarding case selection is presented, including recommendations for application of specific case selection criteria.

In the mid 1960s, an article in *Asha* concerning speech improvement and speech therapy sparked a series of reactions to case selection criteria used in the schools. The first group of respondents were professionals employed in some capacity in a school system. Directors of university training programs contributed to the second article. One question posed in the latter articles was "What guidelines do you use in determining which children whould be enrolled in a clinical speech program?"

Responding to this question, Farquhar identified several factors that she felt should be taken into consideration in case selection (Allen, Black, Burkland, Byrne, Farquhar, Herbert, & Robertson, 1966). One of these was teacher and parental concern regarding the communicative disorder presented by the child and concomitant pressure that might be exerted on him or her. She suggested that a somewhat minor problem could become serious if outside pressures were allowed to continue. With regard to priorities assigned to types of problems, Farquhar recommended that the highest priority be given to stuttering children and those whose communicative disorders were of an organic etiology.

Burkland stressed the importance of maturation in case selection (Allen et al., 1966). Older children presenting problems are less likely to self-correct than are the younger ones; the former, then, should be given priority in case selection.

Allen described a case selection procedure based on test–retest comparisons and subsequent rankings (Allen et al., 1966). In the Kansas City, Missouri schools, kindergarten children were screened each May. The following fall, children previously identified as presenting articulatory disorders were reevaluated and ranked on a 0–5 scale of severity. Children with severe problems (a ranking of 5) were scheduled for therapy, as were children above the first grade level with minor problems.

Robertson reported that the Oakland, Michigan school speech-language pathologists based case load selection on the type of problem presented by the child (Allen et al., 1966). Further, kindergarten children were not included in therapy unless they presented severe problems.

This group of professionals, then, expressed a variety of opinions. Among the factors mentioned were the social effect of the disorder, the influence of maturation, and the type of problem. Similar differences were evident when directors of training programs commented on case selection. Webster, for example, stressed the importance of determining the gap between the child's communicative ability and that which is considered normal (Webster, Perkins, Bloomer, & Pronovost, 1966). She also discussed the mode of testing: conversational speech must be included in any testing procedure in order to obtain an adequate assessment of both articulatory and rhythmic skills. Finally, Webster cautioned that the speech-language pathologist must avoid overevaluating. She warned that the professional should not "try to refine his judgment of the speech problem to the extent that he prolongs diagnosis beyond its usefulness and thus delays therapy; further diagnosis can and does proceed with therapy" (Webster et al., 1966, p. 354). Webster also raised the point that the symptom of the disorder cannot be the only factor on which to base case selection. The social aspects of the problem, its etiology, and the reactions to it must be taken into consideration. She also recommended that the speech-language pathologist consult with others, since he or she observes the child in only one of many settings and other professionals may provide valuable input. After compilation of all available information, the speech-language pathologist may then apply a rating of severity and select those children who need therapy most critically.

According to Perkins, several questions should be answered during the case selection process (Webster et al., 1966). Among these are the following:

- Can the child benefit from public school therapy?
- Does the child require other services (e.g., medical or psychological) more than speech therapy?
- How interfering is the communicative disorder in terms of communication, educational progress, and social adjustment?
- Does the child feel that he or she has a problem and what is his or her reaction to it?
- Is the child mature and motivated enough to benefit from therapy?
- Are the parents and teacher involved with the problem?
- Might the problem persist into adulthood?
- Is scheduling feasible?

Perkins believes that accurate answers to these questions permit efficient case load selection.

Bloomer listed criteria which should be considered in case selection (Webster, 1966). They included the child's age; social aspects of the problem; stimulability; the presence of other developmental problems; the attitudes of the child, of family, and of teachers toward the problem; a familial history of speech disorders; and the length of time the presenting problem has existed.

Speaking specifically of children exhibiting articulatory disorders, Pronovost suggested that several tests be administered to assist the speech-language pathologist in making case selection decisions (Webster et al., 1966). The test battery, recommended only for children who display multiple misarticulations, included the following: an intelligence test, the Carter-Buck Nonsense Syllable Test, a test of auditory discrimination, assessment of diadochokinetic rate, and analysis of a language sample.

A final group of speech-language pathologists addressed the issue of case selection in 1977. Yoder and Stone stressed that children should not be selected on the basis of the number of misarticulations alone (Flower, Leach, Stone, & Yoder, 1967). The specific phonemes in error and the effect of the misarticulations on intelligibility must also be considered. These authors also touched on the area of syntax and suggested that some "articulatory" disorders might actually be syntactic errors. Finally, the authors discussed the necessity of maintaining communication with the classroom teacher about actively participating in the therapy program as well as about those children whose speech differences do not require direct intervention.

Little consensus was found, then, with regard to criteria to be considered in case selection. Professionals working in the field and those involved in training speech-language pathologists have dissimilar ideas regarding the importance of specific factors. As a result, one would anticipate little consistency in case selection techniques among school speech-language pathologists. In general, that is what we find.

A survey of 1462 speech-language pathologists in 1959, for example, revealed that case selection was essentially the responsibility of the individual speech-language pathologist: "Although the clinician usually has someone to whom he is responsible and operates within a framework of established policy...he usually does not need specific administrative approval for the admission of a child into the therapy program" (Bingham et al., 1961, p. 37).

The American Speech-Language-Hearing Association, in an attempt to encourage some uniformity in case selection, described groups of children in need of intervention (American Speech and Hearing Association, 1973–1974). Children to be included in the "communication disorders component" are those with language disorders; chronic vocal disorders; dysfluent speech; hearing impairments that affect social or emotional adjustment and/or educational success; and communicative disorders associated with such conditions as mental retardation, cleft palate, and cerebral palsy. Children presenting these disorders should receive direct intervention. Children in the "communication deviations component" should receive direct or indirect services. Such children exhibit transitory articulatory errors; mild developmental delays in language acquisition; mild hearing impairments; identifiable vocal differences; some misarticulations unrelated to maturation and not affecting intelligibility but possibly causing self-consciousness; mild communicative differences requiring stabilization; and speech and language disorders associated with mental retardation.

Individual states have also provided guidelines for case selection. The North Dakota Department of Public Instruction (1977) suggests a four-stage priority sytem for determining the students for whom direct intervention is appropriate and those for whom indirect services are appropriate.

Although similarities exist between the North Dakota priorities and the ASHA guidelines, the former are more specific and are described in Table 4-2.

The ASHA guidelines have also been expanded for use at the district level. Zemmol (1977) described a priority system of case selection employed in the School District of Ferndale, Michigan. The first priority ranking corresponds

Table 4-2
Intervention Priorities

Priority 1
1. Severe language disorders
2. Complex communicative disorders associated with conditions such as cerebral palsy, mental retardation, cleft palate, or emotional disturbances
3. Unintelligible speech
4. Chronic vocal or fluency disorders
5. Hearing impairments that adversely affect social adjustment or educational success

Priority 2
1. Misarticulation of 4 or more phonemes (but not rated as Priority 1; children in grades 3–12)
2. Moderate language disorders
3. Transitory fluency or vocal problems

Priority 3
1. Consistent misarticulation of 1–3 phonemes (children in grades 3–12)
2. Nonmaturational articulatory errors that do not interfere with intelligibility but may affect self-concept
3. A need for minimal supervision to evaluate carryover
4. Moderate fluency or vocal disorders
5. Language or speech differences that may interfere with overall development

Priority 4
1. Developmental delays in language that should be overcome without intervention
2. Mild articulatory, vocal, or fluency disturbances
3. Mild hearing impairments

SOURCE: North Dakota Department of Public Instruction, 1977.
NOTE: Students who exhibit any one of the listed difficulties are granted the relevant priority.

with the ASHA "communication disorders component" and includes severely handicapped children who require intensive programming. Second priority children ("communication deviations component") present moderate disorders and require less frequent scheduling than first priority students. Students in the third priority group exhibit mild speech or language problems and may be scheduled as feasible. Finally, consultative services are provided.

Although all three sets of guidelines may be helpful, two problems are apparent. With regard to interpretation of the material, What constitutes a mild, moderate, or severe disorder? This is not specified in any of the documents. An even more important question to be asked is whether school speech-language pathologists feel that they need guidelines to assist them in case selection. This question was one of many posed in a 1980 survey of 61 speech-language pathologists working in schools in the United States (Hahn, 1980). The first area explored was determination of what persons or agencies made decisions regarding case selection. Of the 61 respondents, 33 reported professional judgment to be the sole criterion for case selection, 6 cited state regulations, and 2 stated that district regulations governed the process. One respondent indicated that the speech-language supervisor was instrumental in the case selection procedure, and the remaining 19 professionals reported that they were restricted by a combination of state and district regulations and professional judgment. Of the speech-language pathologists functioning under some degree of state-imposed restrictions regarding case selection, 47.37 percent found the regulations to be adequate and helpful, but 31.58 percent indicated that the regulations were too specific. The remaining respondents reported that the regulations were too general to be helpful. When the group without state guidelines was asked whether such regulations were desirable, the overwhelming majority responded negatively; only 22.22 percent favored such guidelines.

Where, then, does this leave the student speech-language pathologist with regard to case selection? The previous discussion illustrated that commonality of thinking among experienced professionals and educators does not exist. Criteria used for case selection range from tangible factors such as the type of problem and the age of the child exhibiting the disorder to less observable components, including the child's reaction to the problem and his or her potential to overcome the deviation without intervention. One might assume that uniformity in case selection methods based on guidelines developed at the district, state, or national levels would be desirable. If, however, the results of Hahn's survey can be generalized, this does not appear to be the wish of practicing speech-language pathologists. They prefer to employ professional judgment rather than conform to regulations, at least at the state level. Since university programs purport to be graduating competent speech-language pathologists who are capable of making judgments regarding etiology and of conducting sensitive evaluations, perhaps it is reasonable that school speech-language pathologists be allowed flexibility in determining which communicatively disordered children should be enrolled for direct intervention and which should receive alternative program management.

MANAGEMENT ALTERNATIVES

Once children with communicative disorders have been identified, diagnosed, and selected for intervention, the speech-language pathologist, in consultation with the parents, teacher, other concerned professionals, and sometimes the child himself or herself, formulates an *individualized education program* (IEP). The preparation of that program is considered in a later chapter. One section of the IEP requires a statement as to which management alternative will best meet the needs of the individual student. In this section of the chapter, intervention options as outlined in the *Standards and Guidelines for Comprehensive Language, Speech, and Hearing Programs in the Schools* are discussed (American Speech and Hearing Association, 1973–1974).

Diagnostic-Educational Team

Some children seen by the speech-language pathologist present problems requiring extensive evaluation by a variety of professional persons. The Diagnostic-Educational Team provides comprehensive assessment by a speech-language pathologist (with expertise in the area of evaluation and with access to numerous diagnostic tools); a physician; a psychologist; and representatives of related disciplines. The purpose of the evaluation is to assist specialists and teachers in designing an educational and support program that will be most appropriate for the child. Children whose primary problem is in the area of speech, language, and/or hearing may be referred as well as children presenting other educational or behavioral disorders.

The functioning of one such team was described by Knight (1974). In St. Louis County, St. Louis, Missouri, children are referred to the Special School District Evaluation Clinic by speech-language pathologists, parents, teachers, or other concerned individuals. Children so referred are then evaluated by a five-member team who assess the child's functioning and study health and family histories. For the language disordered child, Knight reported that team psychologists rely upon the Wechsler Intelligence Scale for Children and the Illinois Test of Psycholinguistic Abilities. Tests administered by the speech-language pathologist may include the Northwestern Syntax Screening Test, the Assessment of Children's Language Comprehension, the Wepman Auditory Discrimination Test, and the Boehm Test of Basic Concepts. Language sampling techniques are employed, and auditory sensitivity is evaluated. Other team members involved are the social worker, who is responsible for interviewing the parents; the educational consultant, who administers formal and informal academic tests; and the consulting pediatrician, who examines the child medically. The findings of this team are transmitted in the form of a recommendation for placement to the program supervisor.

It goes without saying that not all children with speech, hearing, or language disorders will require the services of a diagnostic team. Nevertheless, such a group should be available to evaluate those children presenting complex problems.

Diagnostic Center Placement

Short-term enrollment in a diagnostic center affords the opportunity for children to be thoroughly evaluated and for educational programs to be formulated and assessed. Speech-language pathologists, audiologists, teachers of the hearing impaired, and other specialists are available to provide direct or supportive services to children placed in the center. Again, most students with communicative disorders will not need to be enrolled in such a center, but one should be provided for those students requiring such assessment.

Language Classroom

Young children with serious communicative disorders may be assigned to full-time placement in a language classroom. In that setting, speech-language pathologists provide specialized programs emphasizing language to those students whose disabilities in the area of communication preclude successful placement in the regular classroom.

Since most speech-language pathologists are not specifically trained to function in the classroom, additional preparation is necessary. The transition from itinerant speech-language pathologist to teacher of language disordered children in a self-contained classroom was described by Braunstein and Biederman (1974). Those individuals in preparation for assuming the roles of classroom teachers took coursework in language disabilities, the teaching of reading, and the philosophy of discipline. In addition, they attended workshops and took advantage of other opportunities to increase their understanding of language disorders. In preparing for the personal transition into a classroom setting, Braunstein and Biederman realized that they would have day-long commitments to the children in their classes. Their responsibilites would include everything from collecting lunch money to teaching reading. Nevertheless, their interests in working with language disordered children motivated them to make the adjustments.

A typical daily schedule in a self-contained language classroom demonstrates the emphasis on language. Following the daily opening and preliminary activities, individualized work in reading, math, and spelling is undertaken. Each child has a folder containing his or her daily assignments and when he or she completes a task, another activity may be selected. During this period of independent work, the teacher-clinician is involved with individuals or small groups. Language activities incorporating the academic areas of science and social studies follow lunch and recess. The children are then involved in gross motor activities and, after a story, prepare to go home. Physical education, art and music instruction, and library visits are also planned during the week. It should be noted that capable children are integrated into the regular classroom for portions of the day.

Most language disordered children do not require the intensity that full-time instruction provides. For those students needing such emphasis, however, programming should be provided.

The Transition, or Integration, Class

Children who continue to require special emphasis on language may be placed in the transition, or integration, class. Students in this program spend at least half of each day in the classroom and the remainder of the day in regular rooms. It would appear possible that some children who do not require the intensive instruction provided in the self-contained language class might also benefit from placement in the integration room. Therefore, both children making the transition between the self-contained room and those requiring more language instruction than can be obtained in the resource room may be placed in the integration language class.

The Resource Room

Children with severe speech and/or language disorders may be placed in the Resource Room for less than half of each school day. Here they receive either individual or group therapy for at least one hour daily, while enrolled in regular or special classrooms for the remainder of the day. Resource room placement may be appropriate for children leaving the integration class or for those requiring more intensive work than can be provided supportively.

Crabtree and Peterson (1974) reported on the functioning of speech-language pathologists as resource teachers for children with language-learning disabilities. In this role, the speech-language pathologist must have a sound theoretical background in language development and the ability to analyze and prescribe intervention strategies for children presenting disabilities in phonology, syntax, or semantics. Moreover, according to the authors, the resource teacher must be able to view language, both oral and written, on a continuum and should understand how learning takes place.

Resource room placement, then, might be indicated for children with less serious speech and/or language problems who might not profit from less intensive intervention.

Regular Classroom Placement with Supportive Services

This is the management option that has been utilized with greatest frequency and continues to be employed extensively. Under this model, both direct and indirect supportive services are provided to children with communicative disorders who are enrolled in regular or special classrooms. Services may be delivered on an intensive or intermittent basis, and the speech-language pathologist may be itinerant or assigned to a single school. Chapter 5 deals with scheduling of supportive services.

Hospital or Home Bound

Under special circumstances, communicatively disordered children may be confined to a hospital or to their homes. When this occurs, the only management option available is for the speech-language pathologist to work with the child at the site of confinement.

The Consultant Model

Under any of the management options, the speech-language pathologist may serve as a consultant. In this role, the specialist provides information to classroom teachers when a child or group of children require program modification in order to succeed. The speech-language pathologist might also provide some short-term instruction to children with the understanding that parents and/or teachers will establish maintenance of the desired behavior. In-service training is also the responsibility of the speech-language pathologist functioning in the consultancy model.

Several types of communicative differences may well be served by the consultant. Baskerville (1977) suggested that such a consultant would enhance the Standard English competencies among inner-city children. He points out that nonstandard speech and language patterns among these children are deleterious in terms of educational and vocational success. Teachers, however, are usually not prepared to deal with these communicative differences, and it is reasonable to expect the speech-language pathologist to assist the teachers in developing classroom management strategies. Baskerville suggests that through in-service training, the speech-language pathologist can reinforce the legitimacy of dialectal differences in the minds of the teachers. Additionally, the speech-language pathologist can provide teachers with techniques designed to encourage Standard English usage in the classroom.

Mount (1972) discussed the function of a consultant providing follow-up and aftercare to children seen at a regional diagnostic center. The responsibilities of the consultant were to assist the local speech-language pathologist and the classroom teacher in executing appropriate therapy programs, to provide demonstration therapy, to counsel with parents, and to conduct in-service training programs.

The consultancy model can be adapted to fulfill various needs. It may involve the demonstration of teaching techniques, in-service programming, or preparation of materials designed to meet the special needs of communicatively different students.

Parent–Infant Instruction Services

Speech-language pathologist providing parent–infant instruction are partially involved in the preventive aspect of the profession. In a variety of settings, including the home, the speech-language pathologist provides guidance and information designed to assist parents in encouraging their children to develop appropriate communicative skills. Demonstration teaching may be utilized to show the parents techniques for eliciting speech and language. This model is particularly recommended for children who are considered to be at risk in developing normal learning and communicative skills.

Residential Program Placement

In some instances, the needs of a specific child cannot be met within the regular school setting, and placement in an institution providing special services is required. In other cases, children by reason of inappropriate or delinquent behavior are committed to institutions. When children are placed in state or private schools, the responsibility for providing speech, language, and/or hearing services may be that of the school district or may rest with the institutional personnel. Institutions for delinquent children complying with PL 94-142 also have the responsibility for delivering services to communicatively disordered residents.

Summary of Management Alternatives

It should be apparent to the reader that the speech-language pathologist alone does not determine a child's placement in a program. Although it may be the professional's decision to refer a child to a diagnostic team or to determine that direct or indirect service is preferable, most of the other management alternatives require the consensus of a variety of specialists. In making decisions regarding the placement of a child, all professionals concerned should keep the least restrictive environment concept in mind. A child who can be integrated into the regular classroom for even brief periods of time should be given that opportunity. Even severely handicapped children should spend at least lunch time and recess periods with normally functioning children. If a child can benefit from supportive services alone, then that would be the intervention strategy of preference.

REFERENCES

Allen, E., Black, M., Burkland, M., Byrne, M. C., Farquhar, M. S., Herbert, E. L., & Robertson, M. L. Case selection in the public schools. *Journal of Speech and Hearing Disorders,* 1966, *31,* 157–161.
American Speech and Hearing Association. *Standards and Guidelines for Comprehensive Language, Speech and Hearing Programs in the Schools.* Washington, D.C., 1973–1974.

Baskerville, R. The speech-language pathologist—A resource consultant for enhancing standard english competencies among inner-city children. *Language, Speech, and Hearing Services in Schools,* 1977, *8,* 245–249.

Bingham, D. S., Van Hattum, R. J., Faulk, M. E., & Toussig, E. Program organization and management. *Journal of Speech and Hearing Disorders Monograph Supplement 8,* 1961, 33–49.

Braunstein, S., & Biederman, S. From speech pathologist to language classroom teacher: What does it take? *Language, Speech, and Hearing Services in Schools,* 1974, *5,* 245–252.

Crabtree, M., & Peterson, E. The speech pathologist as a resource teacher for language/learning disabilities. *Language, Speech, and Hearing Services in Schools,* 1974, *5,* 194–197.

Flower, R. M., Leach, E., Stone, C. R., & Yoder, D. E. Case selection. *Journal of Speech and Hearing Disorders,* 1967, *32,* 65–70.

Hahn, C. *An investigation into current procedures of case finding, case selection and scheduling in the schools.* Unpublished M.S. thesis, Southern Illinois University at Edwardsville, 1980.

Hoopes, M., & Dasovich, M. O. Parent counseling: A survey of use by the public school speech clinician. *Journal of the Missouri Speech and Hearing Association,* 1972, *5,* 9–13.

Knight, N. F. Structuring remediation in a self-contained classroom. *Language, Speech, and Hearing Services in Schools,* 1974, *5,* 198–203.

Missouri Special Education Services. *Regulations, Standards and Procedural Guidelines.* Revised. 1977.

Mount, K. H. Speech pathology consultant service in the public school. *Journal of the Missouri Speech and Hearing Association,* 1972, *5,* 17–27.

Neal, W. R. Speech pathology services in the secondary schools. *Language, Speech, and Hearing Services in Schools,* 1976, *7,* 6–16.

North Dakota Department of Public Instruction, *Special Education in North Dakota Guidelines III: Programs for Students with Language, Speech and Hearing Disorders in the Public Schools.* 1977.

O'Toole, T. J., & Zaslow, E. L. Public school speech and hearing programs: Things are changing. *Asha,* 1969, *11,* 499–501.

Sommers, R. K. Case finding, case selection and case load. In R. J. Van Hattum (Ed.), *Clinical speech in the schools.* Springfield: Charles C Thomas Publisher, 1969.

Webster, E. J., Perkins, W. H., Bloomer, H. H., & Pronovost, W. Case selection in the schools. *Journal of Speech and Hearing Disorders,* 1966, *31,* 352–358.

Zemmol, C. S. A priority system of case-load selection. *Language, Speech, and Hearing Services in Schools,* 1977, *8,* 85–98.

5

Scheduling Models

Being realistic, the final system of scheduling selected by the clinician usually represents a compromise between the program which best meets the needs of most of the children and the one that the school environment, administration, and teaching personnel desire and can accommodate. (Van Hattum, 1969, p. 165).

The speech-language pathologist, having completed the case selection procedure, must next schedule those children requiring supportive services, using an appropriate scheduling model. In addition to time allocated for direct therapy, the schedule must permit the speech-language pathologist to execute other duties such as evaluations, conferences, consultations, therapy preparation, and maintenance monitoring. The selection of scheduling models depends upon such variables as the number of schools assigned, the distance between schools, the number of children to be seen, the types of problems presented by the children, and district regulations.

GENERAL CONSIDERATIONS

The initial consideration is the allotment of time for screening and evaluative procedures. In some districts, this may be established for the speech-language pathologist. October 1, for example, may be the deadline for beginning therapy or it may be determined that therapy should be initiated within three weeks after the commencement of school. When guidelines are not available, the speech-language pathologist should allot as much time as is necessary to complete the screening and diagnostic procedure. For example, if the speech-language pathologist services only two schools, each containing two first grades, with a fairly normal distribution of communicative disorders, the screening process might be completed within a week. Depending on the complexity of the disorders presented by the children and the time required to obtain parental permission, evaluative procedures should be accomplished by the end of the second week. The development of individualized education programs (IEPs) and conferences might consume another week, with scheduling done at the completion of these conferences. The latter activities often occur before and after school hours as well as during actual school time. Under these hypothetical circumstances, therapy would begin three weeks after school opened.

Not all screening procedures can be executed so expeditiously. The speech-language pathologist assigned to three or more schools will face different problems, especially if these schools contain rooms for special education children. Ideally, such situations should not exist; that is, speech-language pathologists should not be assigned to service more schools and/or children than they can adequately handle. Unfortunately, this policy is not always enforced. The speech-language pathologist in this situation must function as efficiently as possible. This does not mean that less than adequate attention should be given the screening-evaluative process, but rather that more time must be devoted to it at the expense of early therapeutic intervention. Screening and evaluations under these conditions may take a month to complete, with IEP development and conferences consuming additional time. And screening and diagnostic procedures take more time with young or special education children than with older and/or less involved students. Further, IEP development with multiply handicapped children requires the participation of many professionals, and the logistics of preparation and the IEP conferences may be more time consuming than they are when fewer individuals are involved. Because of these variables, the speech-language pathologist should be allowed to determine the amount of time utilized in pretherapy preparation. When such flexibility is not available, it is the speech-language pathologist's responsibility to, first, adhere to the regulations and second, present evidence to his or her supervisor that will persuade the latter to change the policy.

Although it may seem premature, at the beginning of the year, to establish a date for terminating therapy, many school districts do allow speech-language pathologists to end therapy prior to the closing of school. This permits time for year-end reevaluations, records, reports, and housekeeping chores. In addition, school speech-language pathologists have found that the results of therapy in May and/or early June are not always positive. Field trips, year-end testing, and a variety of extracurricular activities interrupt therapy and may result in a dilution of professional time and energy. These factors combine to encourage the early termination of therapy.

As was true with activities at the outset of school, the speech-language pathologist should be able to decide whether one week is sufficient or whether more time is needed to complete year-end functions. It goes without saying that many duties will be completed outside of school hours: scoring tests, preparing reports, and conferencing with parents may be carried out before or after school. Direct testing, however, must take place during school hours, and an estimate of the amount of time such activities will consume should be made at the beginning of the year.

An approximate schedule for the year, then, should be devised by the speech-language pathologist at the outset. Considering that the typical school year consists of 36 weeks, the following plan may serve as an example. If school opens during the last week of August, it is likely to close at the end of May. Considering again the assignment of two schools with a normal distribution of communicatively disordered children, the speech-language pathologist might anticipate the screening-evaluation-IEP processes to run through the second week in September, with therapy beginning during the third week of that month. Keeping in mind year-end activities, therapy could be terminated at the beginning of May; this would allow two weeks for retesting, report writing, and other closing duties.

This type of schedule has sometimes led to abuses by speech-language pathologists with resultant resentment by classroom teachers. While teachers are spending six hours a day, 36 weeks a year with their children in the classroom, the speech-language pathologist may have one-half day per week without scheduled therapy and only 31 weeks of direct therapy during this same period. There will always be unethical, poorly motivated speech-language pathologists who take advantage of the system. One hopes that there are only a few such people and that the real problem lies in the classroom teachers' lack of understanding of the role and responsibilities of the speech-language pathologist. For example, although the teacher is responsible for the children in a single classroom, the speech-language pathologist is responsible for the majority of children in one or more schools. Further, whereas the classroom teacher may assign "seat work" and have a few minutes from time to time during the day to work on records, the speech-language pathologist is seeing children back-to-back, with no such time available. If teachers, through in-service training, can be made aware of these differences in responsibilities, there is little doubt that they will understand and accept similar differences in scheduling.

Having examined scheduling for the opening and closing of the year, we must now look at scheduling for the week. Historically, speech-language pathologists have been allowed some time each week for coordination activities. These duties include evaluations, parent and/or teacher conferences, record keeping, classroom observations, and related activities. During the author's tenure in the schools, four days were spent in direct scheduled therapy; Friday morning was kept flexible, and Friday afternoon was designated coordination time. Therapy was provided on Friday morning to children needing additional assistance or to those for whom only one-time weekly maintenance therapy was required. During the remainder of the week, children were seen on a twice-weekly basis, receiving therapy on either a Monday–Wednesday or Tuesday–Thursday schedule. Although it was convenient to have the last day of the week flexible, it was probably not a very effective learning strategy. For children receiving therapy on the Monday–Wednesday sequence, four days elapsed between the Wednesday and Monday sessions; the same was true for children on the Tuesday–Thursday schedule. A better model for twice-weekly scheduling would have been Monday–Thursday and Tuesday–Friday, with Wednesday morning kept flexible and the afternoon designated as coordination time. Still not ideal, this arrangement would separate therapy sessions by only three days, rather than four.

A recent survey of school speech-language pathologists attempted to determine the amount of time contemporary professionals have for coordination activities (Hahn, 1980). The results revealed the range to be from no time allotted to six hours (in one day) or more. Approximately 40 percent of the responding speech-language pathologists reported that fewer than 4 hours each week were designated for coordination; an additional 40 percent reported that 4 to 6 hours were set aside. The final 20 percent of the respondents allocated at least one full day for such activities.

It is clear that some time must be allowed for coordination activities. On either an intensive cycle or intermittent schedule, it would appear that a midweek day is preferable. Again, the decision as to whether coordination time is provided, how much time is allowed, and when it occurs may be made by supervisors or administrators. Nevertheless, it would appear that one-half day is the minimum, and one full day is preferable. For purposes of this discussion, Wednesday is designated as the coordination day.

With the yearly schedules established, the school speech-language pathologist must now select a weekly therapy scheduling model. Before we discuss the factors governing selection of such a model, we will examine the major scheduling options.

DESCRIPTIONS OF SCHEDULING MODELS

Intermittent Scheduling

Two basic scheduling models, as well as variations of these models, have been utilized in the school setting: the intermittent model and intensive cycle scheduling. *Intermittent scheduling* involves the establishment of a yearly schedule wherein children are seen a specific number of times each week throughout the academic year. Although some children may be dismissed and others added to the schedule, the school assignments remain the same. The author's own schedule in the schools was alluded to earlier in this chapter; Table 5-1 illustrates this schedule under the heading "Three schools." This schedule accounts for two small schools and one larger school. School A had a higher case load than School B; because morning school sessions were 30 minutes longer than afternoon sessions, School A was scheduled for morning. School C, the largest of the three, received two complete days of therapy. Friday morning was flexible; selected children at School C were seen early, and School B students were serviced in the late morning. Coordination activities consumed Friday afternoons, with the author working out of School C.

In retrospect, this schedule was inefficient. A schedule illustrating a more effective utilization of time appears in Table 5-1 under the heading "Three schools—adjusted."

The speech-language pathologist working in fewer or more than three schools must make appropriate adjustments. Table 5-1 illustrates intermittent scheduling variations based on the number of schools assigned, i.e., one, two, or four schools.

Except in rural areas, it would be highly unusual for a speech-language pathologist to be assigned to more than four schools. In the event that such an assignment were made, it would be necessary to schedule small schools in geographic proximity for either morning or afternoon sessions. Such a schedule is represented in Table 5-1 under the heading "Five schools."

Intermittent scheduling, then, involves the establishment of a schedule that permits children to be seen at least twice weekly throughout the school year. The initial screening and evaluation processes are not necessarily conducted according to the yearly therapy schedule. In other words, the speech-language pathologist will probably complete these activities at one school before moving to another, rather than adhere to the Monday–Thursday, Tuesday–Friday schedule for this portion of his or her yearly work.

Intensive Cycle Scheduling

Intensive cycle scheduling differs from the intermittent model in terms of the number of times per week children are seen and the number of weeks during the year they receive services. In general, on an intensive cycle schedule, students are seen four times each week for a period of at least six weeks and then are furloughed for a specific length of time. The number of therapy blocks during the 36-week school year depends on state or district policies and the number of schools serviced by the individual speech-language pathologist.

Looking again at variations based on the number of schools, the speech-language pathologist assigned to a single building would have the utmost

Table 5-1
Intermittent Schedules

	Monday	Tuesday	Wednesday	Thursday	Friday
Three schools					
A.M.	School A	School C	School A	School C	Schools C, B
P.M.	School B	School C	School B	School C	Coordination office in school C
Three schools—adjusted					
A.M.	School A	School C	Schools B, C	School A	School C
P.M.	School B	School C	Coordination office in school C	School B	School C
One school[a]					
A.M.	Groups 1–8	Groups 17–24	Coordination	Groups 1–8	Groups 17–24
P.M.	Groups 9–16	Groups 25–32	Coordination	Groups 9–16	Groups 25–32
Two schools					
A.M.	School A	School B	Coordination	School A	School B
P.M.	School A	School B	Coordination	School A	School B
Four schools					
A.M.	School A	School C	Coordination	School A	School C
P.M.	School B	School D	Coordination	School B	School D
Five schools					
A.M.	Schools A, B	School D	Coordination	Schools A, B	School D
P.M.	School C	School E	Coordination	School C	School E

[a]This schedule assumes that sessions are 20 minutes in length. The "group" designation is not intended to preclude individual sessions.

flexibility. Screening, evaluations, and IEPs would be completed during the first three or four weeks of school. Assuming that a month was required at the beginning of the year, and also assuming that 2 weeks were set aside for year-end activities, 30 weeks of therapy would be possible. If a strict intensive cycle schedule were employed, the 30 weeks could be divided into 2 8-week blocks and 2 7-week blocks. Since positive results occur early in therapy, the 2 8-week blocks would probably occur first, followed by the 7-week sessions. The result would be the type of schedule illustrated in Table 5-2 for one school. One of the more positive aspects of this schedule is that it does not preclude the provision of intensive therapy throughout the year to those students with complex problems. Combinations of intermittent and intensive cycle service are also possible.

The speech-language pathologist assigned two schools enjoys similar flexibility. Both intensive and intermittent services can be provided according to the needs of the children. One scheduling option is to service School A in the mornings and School B in the afternoons, provided the schools are in close proximity. In order to accommodate kindergarten students in both buildings, the schedule can be reversed during two of the four blocks (Table 5-2).

Another approach to intensive cycle scheduling would be to service School A students for Blocks 1 and 3 and School B children during Blocks 2 and 4 (Table 5-2).

The speech-language pathologist using intensive cycle schedules may not be able to complete screening prior to the intiation of therapy. The North Dakota Department of Public Instruction (1977), for example, presents a block model for four schools in which screening and evaluations for two schools are postponed until therapy is to be started. The allocation of time for this process is unclear. Table 5-3 illustrates that model.

The question of when testing should be scheduled in an intensive cycle model requires some attention. Medical and related referrals should be made expeditiously; in such cases, it is best if all testing and subsequent referrals are accomplished at the beginning of the school year rather than at the beginning of the block. On the other hand, some children with communicative disorders may improve without intervention, and the child presenting a problem in September may not have that same disorder in November. Nevertheless, in order for the speech-language pathologist to plan efficiently for all children with disordered communication, it seems reasonable for all screening, evaluations, and IEPs to be completed prior to the initiation of any therapy.

As noted earlier, it is possible to provide a combination of intensive and intermittent services with some scheduling models. Option 1 of the intensive cycle plan for two schools (Table 5-2) allows for some students to be seen continuously, whereas others may be seen only during specific blocks; therapy for the former children may be either intermittent or intensive. The same flexibility is available when only one school is serviced.

Table 5-2
Intensive Cycle Schedules

	Pretherapy Block (4 weeks)	Block 1 (8 weeks)	Block 2 (8 weeks)	Block 3 (7 weeks)	Block 4 (7 weeks)	Posttherapy Block (2 weeks)
One school	Screening, evaluations, IEP development, and scheduling	Group 1 students	Group 2 students	Group 1 students	Group 2 students	Year-end duties
Two schools: Option 1	Screening, evaluations, IEP development, and scheduling	School A (A.M.) School B (P.M.)	School B (A.M.) School A (P.M.)	School A (A.M.) School B (P.M.)	School B (A.M.) School A (P.M.)	Year-end duties
Two schools: Option 2	Screening, evaluations, IEP development, and scheduling	School A	School B	School A	School B	Year-end duties

Table 5-3
Block Scheduling for Four Schools

Testing	Block 1 (8–9 weeks)	Testing	Block 2 (8–9 weeks)	Block 3 (8–9 weeks)	Block 4 (8–9 weeks)
Schools A and B	Schools A and B	Schools C and D	Schools C and D	Schools A and B	Schools C and D

SOURCE: North Dakota Department of Public Instruction, 1977. Reprinted by permission.

DISCUSSION OF SCHEDULING MODELS

Having described some of the scheduling models available to the speech-language pathologist, some consideration of the relative merit and utilization of these systems is appropriate. An early reference to scheduling systems appeared in 1956. Fein, Golman, Kone, and McClintock (1956) described problems encountered in the Chicago schools where each speech-language pathologist was responsible for an average of five schools. At that time, the school speech-language pathologist visited each school once weekly. The block system was rejected as administratively unwieldy in such a large system (70 speech-language pathologists were employed at that time), and a modified plan was initiated. The system this plan outlined allowed the speech-language pathologist to provide twice-weekly therapy to children in one group of schools during the first semester and to children in the other group of schools during the second semester. The question to be answered was whether this service delivery system would be more efficient than the provision of services once per week during the entire academic year. An experimental group and a control group of children served as subjects. A total of 299 children received therapy twice weekly for one semester (experimental group) only, and a like number received therapy one time per week from September through June. At the end of one academic year, the results showed little difference in improvement between the two groups of children. It was determined that the needs, interests, and convenience of the individual schools and speech-language pathologists should determine which scheduling model was selected.

McDonald and Frick (1957) reviewed factors that should be considered in choosing a scheduling model and concluded that flexibility, rather than ridigity, was the key. They suggested that intensive cycle scheduling might allow for such flexibility in the school setting and encouraged the school speech-language pathologist to experiment with the block and other systems rather than adhere strictly to an intermittent schedule.

During the 1958–1959 school year, the Arlington County Public School speech-language pathologists instituted a research project to compare the effectiveness of the block and traditional methods of scheduling (Ervin, 1965). The subjects were 102 second and third grade students with articulatory disorders. Half of the children were assigned to the experimental group, and matched subjects were placed in the control group. Control group subjects received therapy in half-hour sessions, twice each week, for 20 weeks. Children in the experimental group received a half-hour of therapy four days each week for two five-week blocks; one block occurred in the fall and the other in the spring. Both groups of children had at least 34 therapy sessions during the year. The results of the study supported the effectiveness of the block system of scheduling children with articulatory disorders; children receiving intensive therapy evidenced more improvement than those receiving intermittent help. The author cautioned, however, that similar results might not occur if the block were employed with children presenting other types of communicative disorders.

In an early-1960 survey, speech-language pathologists, local supervisors, and state supervisors were asked to compare the effectiveness of block and traditional scheduling systems (Bingham, Van Hattum, Faulk, & Toussig, 1961). Although there appeared to be some confusion about what a "block" system was, it was found that the majority of the speech-language pathologists (81 percent) and local supervisors (70 percent) had never employed intensive cycle scheduling. Of the state supervisors, 33 percent had not used the block system either. Those who had had experience with intensive cycle scheduling appeared to favor the traditional system.

Because of the confusion created by the original survey, a follow-up questionnaire was distributed to 100 speech-language pathologists. Of the 75 responding to the survey, 10 did not know what a block system was. The remaining 65 speech-language pathologists, when asked to describe a block schedule, provided 26 variations of the system. This continued confusion over terminology led the investigators to question the validity of both questionnaires.

Weaver and Wollershein (1963) reported on a pilot study comparing block and intermittent scheduling systems. The research hypothesis was that children with articulatory disorders would benefit more from intensive cycle scheduling than from intermittent services. The experimental group, comprised of 158 students, received intensive therapy; 243 control children received intermittent services. Those on the block were seen four times each week during each of the three five-week blocks; during the off-service block, children were seen once each week. Control group children received therapy twice weekly for the entire year or until they were dismissed. At the end of the year, all children were reevaluated, and it was found that children on the block system made more progress than those receiving intermittent services. Moreover, the experimental group made these gains in fewer minutes of therapy. The researchers expressed strong support for intensive cycle scheduling with children presenting articulatory disorders.

Black (1972) described a unique intensive cycle scheduling model in which children did not miss specific classes each day in order to attend therapy. Under this system, a child was seen on Monday at 1:00 P.M., on Tuesday at 1:20 P.M., on Wednesday at 1:40 P.M. and so forth. Although this would seem to create serious problems in therapy attendance, Black reported that teachers supported this staggered system. With regard to the results of intensive cycle therapy, a doubled dismissal rate was reported. Of the children enrolled under the intermittent system, 17 percent were dismissed during or at the end of the year, whereas 34 percent was the dismissal rate under the block system. The author concluded that intensive cycle scheduling facilitates positive results, especially when applied to children with articulatory disorders.

The same sort of staggered schedule was employed by Strong (1973). Although Strong expressed satisfaction with the block, her question related to teacher reaction to the system. A questionnaire was sent to participating teachers in two schools; 27 teachers responded to the survey. Although in many instances the teachers noted little difference between the block and intensive cycle schedules, they did show a preference for the former. The author cited ease of scheduling, fewer absences, and better carry-over from session to session among the positive aspects of the block system. Disadvantages included room availability and the effect of extended absences of the speech-language pathologist on the therapy program at a specific school.

An ASHA task force reviewed intermittent and intensive cycle scheduling in the early 1970s ("American Speech and Hearing Assocation Task Force Report," 1973). They reported that traditional scheduling is simple and convenient but that the speech-language pathologist should determine whether this model meets the needs of all communicatively disordered children. Regarding intensive cycle scheduling, the task force cited the higher dismissal rate for students with articulatory disorders as an advantage. They noted better carry-over from session to session, more opportunities for the speech-language pathologist to interact with school personnel, and a reduction of travel time as additional advantages. It was remarked that the intensive cycle schedule is not as effective for children with organically based disorders, severe functional problems, or language disabilities.

Weston and Harber (1975) reported results from intensive cycle scheduling that conflict with those obtained in earlier studies. In this study, the paired stimuli technique was employed with 70 children presenting articulatory disorders. The subjects were placed in one of five groups: Group I students attended therapy on Monday, Wednesday, and Friday; Group II attended on Tuesday and Thursday; Group III attended on Monday and Wednesday; Group IV attended on Monday, Tuesday, Thursday, and Friday; and Group V attended on Monday, Tuesday, and Friday. Group III students were the first to reach the criterion established by the paired stimuli program; it took these children a mean time of 42.86 minutes. Group II children reached criterion in a mean time of 73.64 minutes. Interestingly enough, the students attending therapy four times weekly required the most time to attain criterion: their mean time was 138.21 minutes. The authors cautioned that these results cannot be generalized to children displaying other types of communicative disorders nor to students with articulatory disorders when a systematic program is not applied. Nevertheless, the authors' findings suggest that intensive therapy is not required when the paired stimuli technique is utilized.

The comparable effectiveness of intensive cycle and intermittent therapy remains unclear. Although the results of most studies indicate that block systems are more effective with children displaying articulatory disorders, the Weston and Harber investigation is not consistent with this finding. Moreover, evidence does not exist to suggest that intensive cycle scheduling is effective with children presenting other types of communicative disorders.

One final question relates to the current utilization of intensive cycle and intermittent scheduling systems. Hahn (1980) in a recent nationwide survey, found that the intermittent system was employed by the overwhelming majority of responding speech-language pathologists. Only 8.33 percent reported using an intensive cycle schedule, whereas approximately 35 percent employed other methods and 3.57 percent utilized both intensive cycle and intermittent systems. The remaining speech-language pathologists employed traditional scheduling. It would appear, therefore, that the intermittent scheduling model continues to enjoy popularity over block systems.

FACTORS GOVERNING SCHEDULING

The ASHA Task Force on Scheduling identified 10 factors that should be considered before a scheduling model is selected ("American Speech and Hearing Association Task Force Report," 1973). Although these factors relate specifically to the number of children who can be enrolled in therapy at one time, they are also pertinent in determining which system is appropriate in a given situation.

Initially, the Task Force suggested that the criteria for case selection will influence the number of children who can be enrolled as well as the choice of scheduling model. It is assumed that more liberal case selection procedures would decrease case load size and increase the speech-language pathologist's options in selecting a scheduling model.

An important consideration is the geographic location of the schools assigned to the speech-language pathologist. If he or she is to service several rural schools that are not in close proximity, and if each school contains relatively few communicatively disordered children, the case load size will be reduced and the scheduling models restricted. This situation does not lend itself well to intensive cycle scheduling.

The types of communicative disorders presented by the children as well as the severity of these problems will influence the selection of a scheduling model. Previously discussed research has indicated that children displaying functional articulatory disorders may improve more under an intensive cycle system than under intermittent scheduling. When the speech-language pathologist's case load consists chiefly of children with articulatory disorders, some variation of the block system may be appropriate. Since it appears, however, that case load distribution is changing, and since the efficacy of block scheduling for children with other types of communicative disorders is questionable, it would seem that intermittent scheduling or a combination of intermittent and intensive cycle scheduling would best meet the needs of such students.

The Task Force suggested that school codes and transportation regulations might prevent the provision of services in a centralized location. Nevertheless, the speech-language pathologist assigned to five rural schools might, if district policies permitted, work out of one school with children in need of services transported to that location. This arrangement would allow the speech-language pathologist to service more children by reducing travel time. It would also permit greater scheduling flexibility.

The number and size of the schools serviced must be considered in scheduling. The speech-language pathologist assigned to a single school or to two buildings has the opportunity to select a scheduling model appropriate to the needs of the children. As the number of schools increases, travel time must be considered, and the scheduling options are reduced.

The availability of other staff members who might assume some of the speech-language pathologist's responsibilities will influence the number of children who may be accommodated. School secretaries, public health nurses, and paraprofessionals may be among those individuals. Secretaries may assist by retrieving and by typing materials and reports. In some districts, public health officials are responsible for hearing screenings; when this is the case, the speech-language pathologist may not be required to participate. Finally, the utilization of supportive personnel could permit the professional to service more children. In addition to preparing therapy materials, the paraprofessional might also monitor student progress or administer selected therapy programs. When such assistance is available, more children can be serviced and more intensive therapy provided. Again, the speech-language pathologist will have greater flexibility in selecting a scheduling model.

One scheduling decision that will influence the number of children who can be serviced at any given time is whether individual or group sessions are to be provided. The issue of which service delivery technique facilitates the modification of communicative disorders has been a controversial one. Some professionals have advocated individual therapy, suggesting that group work is a waste of both student and professional time. Mowrer (1972), for example, discussed group vs. individual therapy in terms of cost accounting. He pointed out that children seen twice weekly in a group of four spend three times more time listening than they do responding. Assuming that each session is 20 minutes in length and that therapy time is divided equally among the four children, each child would spend 10 minutes each week in direct interaction with the speech-language pathologist and 30 minutes listening to the other children respond. Since some research suggests that listening does little to change speech behavior, Mowrer contends that group therapy is inefficient with children.

Special education policies in North Dakota are consistent with Mowrer's position on group therapy (North Dakota Department of Public Instruction, 1977). Because the modification of oral communication disorders requires verbal practice by the child and feedback from the speech-language pathologist, it is recommended that individual therapy be provided. Exceptions occur when group participation is an inherent part of the therapy program, as it might be with language disordered children or students who stutter.

Not all professionals agree that individual therapy is preferable. There are those who suggest that group therapy is a waste of time only when the speech-language pathologist is not skilled in handling groups. Most would concur that children with language disorders benefit from group participation and that students who stutter profit from interaction with children with similar problems. Proponents of group therapy say that it can be equally beneficial for children with articulatory and vocal problems. Regarding articulatory disabilities, it is possible to group children with similar or dissimilar phonemic errors. When the latter is done, children in the group may serve as models and monitors for each other. In this way, they become acive group participants rather than passive observers. When children are properly grouped according to age and sex—and possibly disorder—and when the speech-language pathologist is trained to handle groups, this technique can be effective. If the children are grouped for the convenience of the speech-language pathologist or the classroom teacher, or if the speech-language pathologist provides individual therapy in a group situation, then group therapy lacks efficacy.

It is often supposed that more children can be handled by the speech-language pathologist if group therapy is employed. Although it appears that the ASHA Task Force regarded this to be the case, the effect of group or individual therapy on scheduling is directly tied to the next factor, the length and number of sessions conducted during the day. Assuming that the typical school day is six hours in length, the speech-language pathologist should have the opportunity to schedule according to the needs of the students. Individual sessions should be a minimum of 15 minutes; group sessions may be 20–30 minutes in length. For the purposes of this discussion, the assumption is made that individual sessions last 15 minutes and group sessions last 30 minutes. Employing a strict schedule of individual therapy, 24 children could be seen each day and thus 48 children serviced on a twice-weekly intermittent system. Such a case load would be manageable if the children presented a normal distribution of communicative disorders. Using a group scheduling model with four children in each group, a total of 48 children could be seen daily with a case load of 96. Since it would be unusual for each group to be that large, a more reasonable case load estimate might be in the neighborhood of 80–85. Depending on the complexity of the communicative disorders presented by the children, the latter may or may not be a manageable number.

It is seen that employment of group scheduling provides less therapy for more children. When such scheduling meets the needs of the students, it is appropriately applied. For the most part, however, it is more reasonable to combine group and individual sessions throughout the day. Children with articulatory and linguistic disorders may be grouped together, and students with fluency or vocal disorders may be involved in a combination of group and individual sessions. The number and length of sessions are also related to the types and complexity of the problems presented by the children. As noted in previous discussions, there is little evidence that children possessing other than articulatory disorders benefit from intensive cycle scheduling. Therefore, regardless of the speech-language pathologist's preference for group of individual sessions or the selection of a time frame for conducting these sessions, if the case load includes children with language, vocal, or fluency disorders, then intermittent or a combination of intensive cycle and intermittent scheduling should be employed.

The final two factors cited by the task force include coordination time and time allocated for other responsibilities. Since these variables were discussed earlier in this chapter, additional consideration would be redundant.

These, then, are the factors that should be considered in the selection of a scheduling model. Although each one of the variables is important, the reader is aware that the most critical factor relates to the needs of the individual children. The ideal schedule is one that is flexible and offers opportunities for both intensive and intermittent service delivery designed to meet such needs.

REFERENCES

American Speech and Hearing Association task force report on traditional scheduling procedures in schools. *Language, Speech, and Hearing Services in Schools,* 1973, *4,* 100–109.

Bingham, D. S., Van Hattum, R. J., Faulk, M. E., & Toussig, E. Program organization and management. *Journal of Speech and Hearing Disorders Monograph Supplement 8,* 1961, 33–49.

Black, M. E. Happenings in speech correction. *The Illinois Speech and Hearing Journal,* 1972, *5,* 22–24.

Ervin, J. C. The effectiveness of block scheduling versus cycle scheduling for articulation therapy for grades two and three in the public schools. *Journal of Speech and Hearing Association* (State of Virginia), Spring 1965, 7–13.

Fein, B. G., Golman, M. G., Kone, H. J., & McClintock, C. R. Effective utilization of staff time in public school speech correction. *Journal of Speech and Hearing Disorders,* 1956, *21,* 283–291.

Hahn, C. An investigation into current procedures of case finding, case selection, and scheduling in the schools. Unpublished M.S. thesis, Southern Illinois University at Edwardsville, 1980.

McDonald, E. T., & Frick, J. V. The frequency and duration of treatment sessions in speech correction. *Journal of Speech and Hearing Disorders,* 1957, *22,* 724–728.

Mowrer, D. E. Accountability and speech therapy in the public schools. *Asha,* 1972, *14,* 111–115.

North Dakota Department of Public Instruction. *Special education in North Dakota guidelines III: Programs for students with language, speech and hearing disorders in the public schools.* 1977.

Strong, P. A. Try the block: you may like it: classroom teachers do. *The Illinois Speech and Hearing Journal,* 1973, *7,* 18–20.

Van Hattum, R. J. *Clinical speech in the schools.* Springfield: Charles C Thomas, Publisher, 1969.

Weaver, J. B, & Wollersheim, J. P. A pilot study comparing the block system and the intermittent system of scheduling speech correction cases in the public schools. Champaign, Illinois: Champaign Community Unit 4 Schools, 1963.

Weston, A. J., & Harber, S. K. The effects of scheduling on progress in paired-stimuli articulation therapy. *Language, Speech, and Hearing Services in Schools,* 1975, *6,* 96–101.

6

Individualized Education Programs

As we look for ways to comply with the IEP regulations, let us not forget that all educational personnel are equal partners in the enterprise and that we are accountable for out efforts not only to handicapped pupils, their parents, and the public, but to each other as well. (Reynolds, 1978, p. 62).

Consistent with the mandate of PL 94-142, the school speech-language pathologist must prepare an *individualized education program* (IEP) for each communicatively disordered child in the case load. Although preprofessional and master's level students in speech-language pathology are required to write session plans using behavioral language, the IEP format may not be familiar.

FEDERAL IEP REGULATIONS

Section 4 of PL 94-142 defines an IEP as follows:

The term 'individualized education program' means a written statement for each handicapped child developed in any meeting by a representative of the local educational agency or an intermediate educational unit who shall be qualified to provide, or supervise the provision of, specially designed instruction to meet the unique needs of handicapped children, the teacher, the parents or guardian of such child, and, whenever appropriate, such child, which statement shall include (A) a statement of the present levels of educational performance of such child, (B) a statement of annual goals, including short-term instructional objectives, (C) a statement of the specific educational services to be provided to such child, and the extent to which such child

89

will be able to participate in regular educational programs, (D) the projected date for initiation and anticipated duration of such services, and (E) appropriate objective criteria and evaluation procedures and schedules for determinining, on at least an annual basis, whether instructional objectives are being achieved. (PL 94-142, 1975).

The law, then, requires the speech-language pathologist to (1) describe the presenting problem, (2) project objectives and goals for the year, (3) determine which service delivery option will best meet the child's needs, (4) anticipate the length of time it will take the child to reach the goals, and (5) describe the methods by which progress will be measured. Although the legal language may appear to make the requirements more complex, the law demands little more than the student in training is asked to do. The seemingly difficult requirement is the development of the IEP. This is a group project rather than one completed by the speech-language pathologist working in isolation. Participants include the parents and may involve other professionals and the child. The major responsibility for program development resides with the professional, but parental participation should provide the speech-language pathologist with additional insight into the individual child's abilities and disabilities. As an added benefit, involvement of the parents in IEP planning should increase their participation in program implementation. Similarly, when children can take part in the IEP planning, their roles in the habilitative effort are more clearly defined. Although the IEP is not a legal contract, all individuals involved in program development agree to the appropriateness of these goals and procedures and assume responsibility for the execution of the plan.

In the ensuing discussion, it is apparent that individual states have expanded on the legal requirements for IEPs.

STATE IEP REGULATIONS

Illinois is one state that has provided guidelines for the development of IEPs and the IEP process (State Board of Education et al., 1979). This process is illustrated in Figure 6-1. The initial responsibility of the local district, as illustrated in the flow chart, is public notification of the annual screening. It is required that all exceptional children between the ages of 3 and 21 be identified and that residents within the district be informed of the rights of exceptional children and of programming available for these students. The screening process includes assessment of preschool children as well as speech and language screening of all children entering public school programs. Following screening, or upon the recommendation of parents, agencies, or professional persons, children may be referred for case study evaluations. The school district determines whether a case study evaluation should be conducted or if outside services should be sought and notifies the parents of this decision. This written notification must be in the parents' native language and must include an explanation of procedural safeguards, a description of the proposed action, and information on procedural safeguards. Before proceeding with the case study evaluation, written parental consent must be obtained. If the parents do not agree to such an evaluation, a due process hearing may be requested by the district. Figure 6-2 illustrates a formal request to evaluate a child.

Once parental consent is secured, the case study evaluation is planned. Children whose problems appear to be limited to speech and language must be screened for hearing sensitivity, and their medical and academic histories and current functioning must be reviewed. In addition, a certified speech-language pathologist must interview each child and assess his speech and language competencies. Following the case study evaluation, the speech-language pathologist determines the child's need and eligibility for services and convenes an IEP conference. Figure 6-3 illustrates notification to the parents of the time and date for the IEP meeting. After this meeting, recommendations are made to the local district superintendent or his representative regarding placement of the child, and the IEP is implemented.

Children presenting multiple disorders require a comprehensive case study evaluation. In addition to the information obtained on the child with a suspected speech and/or language disorder, the following must be done: consultation with parents, compilation of a social history, vision screening, assessment of the learning environment, and any special evaluations that may be necessary. The latter may include psychological assessment, medical examination, and/or audiological testing. All evaluations must be done at the expense of the local school district; if the parents object to any part of the assessment, the district is financially obligated to cover the cost of an independent evaluation. Once the results of the case study evaluation have been reviewed, a multidisciplinary and/or IEP conference must be convened. Parents must be informed of this meeting and invited to attend and participate. During such conferences, the participants review their findings in order to establish a composite understanding of the child's behavior. In addition, the child's eligibility for services, his or her educational needs, and the most appropriate special placement are determined. Recommendations are then made regarding the child's placement in the least restrictive educational environment close to the child's home. A written report of the conference must be prepared and filed and the parents must be informed that they may have access to this report.

In the event that the multidisciplinary and IEP conference are not combined, an additional meeting must be held to prepare the IEP. This conference should be convened within 30 days after the child's need for special services has been identified. Participants in this meeting should include a district representative, the child's teacher, the child's parents or guardians

92

Figure 6-1. Individualized education program (IEP) process. Redrawn from State Board of Education et al., 1979. Courtesy of Illinois Office of Education.

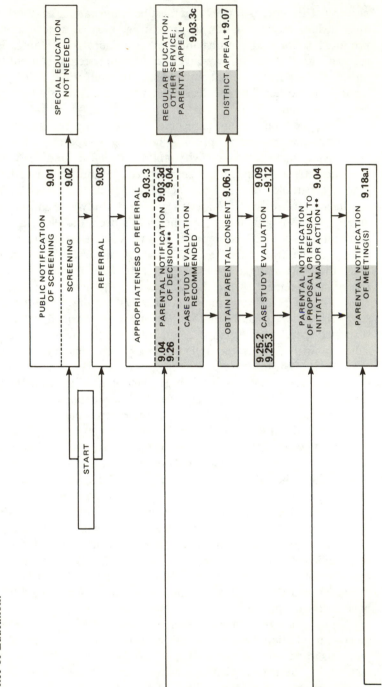

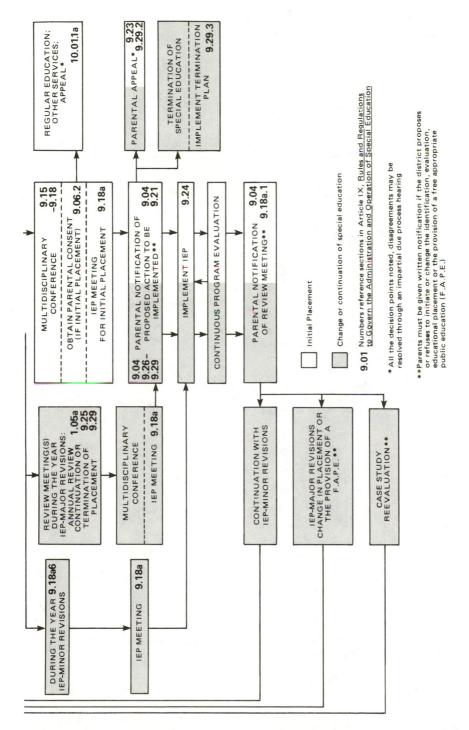

MULTIDISCIPLINARY CONFERENCE **9.15 –9.18**

OBTAIN PARENTAL CONSENT (IF INITIAL PLACEMENT) **9.06.2**

IEP MEETING FOR INITIAL PLACEMENT **9.18a**

REGULAR EDUCATION; OTHER SERVICES: APPEAL* **10.01.1a**

PARENTAL NOTIFICATION OF PROPOSED ACTION TO BE IMPLEMENTED** **9.04 9.21**

PARENTAL APPEAL* **9.23 9.29.2**

TERMINATION OF SPECIAL EDUCATION

IMPLEMENT TERMINATION PLAN **9.29.3**

IMPLEMENT IEP **9.24**

CONTINUOUS PROGRAM EVALUATION

PARENTAL NOTIFICATION OF REVIEW MEETING** **9.04 9.18a.1**

REVIEW MEETING(S) DURING THE YEAR IEP-MAJOR REVISIONS: ANNUAL REVIEW CONTINUATION OR TERMINATION OF PLACEMENT **1.05a 9.25 9.29**

MULTIDISCIPLINARY CONFERENCE

IEP MEETING **9.18a**

9.04 9.26– 9.29

DURING THE YEAR **9.18a6** IEP-MINOR REVISIONS

IEP MEETING **9.18a**

CONTINUATION WITH IEP-MINOR REVISIONS

IEP-MAJOR REVISIONS CHANGE IN PLACEMENT OR THE PROVISION OF A F.A.P.E.**

CASE STUDY REEVALUATION**

☐ Initial Placement

▨ Change or continuation of special education

9.01 Numbers reference sections in Article IX, Rules and Regulations to Govern the Administration and Operation of Special Education

* All the decision points noted, disagreements may be resolved through an impartial due process hearing

** Parents must be given written notification if the district proposes or refuses to initiate or change the identification, evaluation, educational placement or the provision of a free appropriate public education (F.A.P.E.)

93

```
_____                    RE:_____
          (Speech Pathologist)
SCHOOL:_____                    D.O.B.:_____
DATE:_____                    I.D.#:_____
```

Dear Parent:

On _____, _____ filed a referral requesting that
your child be evaluated by this office. We intend to proceed with an individual Speech
and Language case study evaluation of your child for the following reason(s):_____
_____
_____

With your permission, the evaluation procedures we may use with your child to assist us in
planning an appropriate therapy program are as follows:

> An assessment of your child's speech and language.
> A review of your child's medical history and current health status.
> An interview with your child.
> A hearing screening.
> A review of your child's academic history and current educational functioning.
> A consultation with you if needed.

This evaluation and subsequent parent conference(s) will be completed within sixty (60) school days of the date of
receipt of the signed permission. You will be informed in writing as to the date, time, and location of this conference.
Your child will not receive speech and language therapy services without your knowledge.

Please be advised that according to the Rules and Regulations to Govern the Administration and Operation of Special
Education (filed pursuant to Chapter 122, Article XIV, Illinois Revised Statutes, 1975) you have the right to object to
the proposed evaluation of your child. If you object to the proposed evaluation of your child, we would like to discuss
this with you within thirty (30) days. During this period you have the right to meet with the Department Supervisor,
the school principal, your child's teacher, and myself to try to alleviate your objections. If after an informal
conference we cannot come to a mutual acceptance of the proposed evaluation, you are advised that the Peoria Public
Schools, District #150, may request an impartial due process hearing.

You are also advised that you have the right to review all records related to the reason for the evaluation, know the
results of the evaluation, and participate in the conference(s) at which the speech and language therapy plan for your
child will be developed. Additionally, you have the right to obtain an independent speech and language evaluation from
a clinically certified speech pathologist.

Following is a Permission Form which is to be completed by you and returned to me within ten
(10) school days. Should you have any questions please do not hesitate to call me. Return
all copies of this form to me at _____ School.

                                               Sincerely,

                                               _____ 672-_____
                                               (Speech Pathologist)   Phone
----

I am in receipt of the Intent and Procedures to conduct a Speech and Language evaluation of
my child,_____. I have been informed of my rights and know that
my child will not receive Speech and Language therapy services without my knowledge. I
understand the reasons and the description of the evaluation process that you have provided
and have checked the appropriate box below.

> YES ☐ Permission is given to conduct the Speech and Language evaluation.
> NO ☐ Permission is denied.

Parent/Guardian Signature:_____ Date:_____

D.O.C.: w/Master File, y/Sp. P., p/Parent, g/Sp. P.
Rev.: 04-80

Figure 6-2. Peoria Public Schools, District 150, Special Services Division, Form S/L
#2. Courtesy of Peoria Public Schools.

_____
(Speech Pathologist)

DATE:_____

RE:_____
D.O.B.:_____
I.D.#:_____

Dear Parent:

The speech and language evaluation of your child has been completed. As a result of this evaluation, it has been determined that your child would benefit from speech and language therapy. Before this support service can begin, it is important that you be informed of the results of the evaluation and to participate in the development of your child's Individual Educational (Therapy) Program (IEP). We would like to meet with you to discuss the evaluation and to assist in the preparation of the therapy program on:

_____, _____, at _____ at _____
      (Day)   (Date)   (Time)   (School)

Check the appropriate box(s), sign and date below. Please return all copies to me within ten (10) school days. If you should have any questions, please call me.

                                        Sincerely,

                                                            672-
                                        _____
                                        (Speech Pathologist)   Phone
----

YES ☐   I can keep this appointment.

NO ☐   I cannot keep this appointment, but

        YES ☐   I give my permission for my child to receive speech and language services
                and for you to develop my child's Individual Educational Program (IEP).
                By giving my permission without a conference, I understand that all
                papers relevant to the evaluation, including actual results of the assess-
                ment are available for my inspection, the records pertaining to this eval-
                uation are available to me for copying, and my child's IEP will be sent to me.

        NO ☐   I do not give my permission for my child to receive speech and language
                services and for you to develop my child's IEP.

Please be advised that according to the Rules and Regulation to Govern the Administration and Operation of Special Education (filed pursuant to Chapter 122, Article XIV, Illinois Revised Statutes, 1975) you have the right to object to the proposed support service which is being recommended for your child. If within ten (10) school days you object to the proposed support service we would like to meet with you sometime during the next 30 days. During this period you have the right to meet with us to try to resolve any differences. If we cannot resolve any disagreement informally you have the right to request a hearing before an impartial officer. If you decide to request a hearing you will need to write a letter to Mr. Harry F. Whitaker, Superintendent, Peoria Public Schools. This letter shall specifically request a District level hearing with an impartial hearing officer and shall describe the reason(s) the hearing is being requested and shall provide all other information pertinent to the request.

You are also advised that you have the right at your expense, to the following: to be represented by legal counsel, bring witnesses, request certain school personnel to be present, cross examine, obtain an independent evaluation, request an open hearing.

If the child has not reached the age of majority, you have the right to determine if the child shall attend the hearing, except on a finding by the hearing officer that attendance would be harmful to the welfare of the child. The child may then be excluded from all or part of the hearing. The burden of proof as to the adequacy and appropriateness of the proposed course of action shall be upon the school district. A tape recording or other verbatim record of the hearing shall be made and shall be controlled by the Illinois State Board of Education. You shall have the right to a copy of this record on request. At all stages of the hearing, interpretation for the deaf and interpreters in the primary language of the home (when other than English) shall be provided at public expense. During any period of disagreement over placement, your child will continue in his present educational placement.

If you do not grant permission and we cannot resolve any disagreement through an informal conference and you do not request a hearing, be advised that the Peoria Public Schools may proceed with the proposed support service(s).

Signature, Parent/Guardian: _____ Date:_____

D.O.C.: w/Master File, y/Sp.P., p/Parent, g/Sp.P.   Phone:_____
REV.: 04-80

Figure 6-3. Peoria Public Schools, District 150, Special Services Division, Form S/L #3. Courtesy of Peoria Public Schools.

and, when appropriate, the child; other persons may be invited by the parents or local district officials. If the parents cannot attend the meeting, other opportunities for participation must be provided. During the IEP meeting, placement of the child in the most appropriate environment is considered, short-term objectives and long range goals are established, and evaluative criteria are outlined.

The child's parents must be notified in writing of the results of the case study evaluation, the proposed placement, and the services to be delivered 10 calendar days before the child is to be placed in a special program. The parents must also be informed of their right to object to this proposal and notified that they have 10 calendar days in which to appeal the placement. If no objection is made, the IEP is implemented as soon as possible or at least by the beginning of the next school semester. Interim services must be provided to the child awaiting placement.

Once the child has been placed in the appropriate educational environment, continuous evaluation of progress is recommended. Illinois rules and regulations mandate that an annual review of short-term objectives be completed, but this review should be supplemented by periodic monitoring of progress so that the appropriateness of the IEP may be evaluated. Although revisions in the IEP may be made at any time by convening an IEP meeting, formal annual reviews are required. Again, parents are notified of the review conferences, and all professionals involved with the child are invited to participate. During this meeting, the child's current functioning is reviewed as it relates to the objectives set forth in the IEP. In some cases, additional evaluations may be recommended and the IEP may be revised. When the child no longer requires services, special education is terminated. Again, a conference is held and parental participation is encouraged.

As is apparent in Figure 6-1, multiple options are available for the entry IEP meetings. Similarly, opportunities for parental and district appeal, revisions of the IEP, and reevaluation of the child are provided throughout the IEP process. In this discussion, only the general sequence of the process recommended by the State of Illinois has been presented. Students and professionals in other states must consult district and state guidelines for specific IEP procedures. It should be noted that the speech-language pathologist working with a child whose only disability is in the area of oral communication assesses the child, determines the need and eligibility for services, and then convenes the IEP conference. After its cooperative development, the IEP is implemented by the speech-language pathologist. The state requires annual review meetings, and the speech-language pathologist is obligated to provide continuous monitoring of progress.

The State of North Dakota has also developed policies based on the requirements of PL 94-142 (North Dakota Department of Public Instruction, 1977). Their student evaluation procedures begin with the screening process, for which parental consent is not required. Suspect students may then receive additional screenings or may be observed in a variety of situations, still without parental approval, before a decision is made to proceed with formal testing. (Although this may be the practice in Illinois, provision for such intermediate screening is not specified in the rules and regulations.) Once written permission is obtained from the parents, formal testing can be done on those children requiring such evaluation. With regard to speech and/or language disorders, the North Dakota guidelines recommend that formal or informal procedures be employed in each area of communication identified as defective by the screening. Written reports of the evaluation must be sent to the principal, superintendent, or director of special education; the speech-language pathologist retains a copy of this report. Prior to the implementation of therapy, a conference is held to approve a preliminary IEP. Participants include the parents, principal, and appropriate special education personnel. Within 30 days after the child has been enrolled in a special education program, a comprehensive IEP must be prepared and reviewed by the parents. Illinois regulations, on the other hand, specify that the formal IEP must be approved prior to enrollment in a special program. Annual reviews are required in North Dakota, as is parental approval of all IEP revisions.

The policies of these two states are in conformity with PL 94-142 but do present some procedural differences. Access to the rules and regulations of other states would probably reveal similar differences in adherence to the federal law.

IEP DEVELOPMENT

Although many attempts have been made to provide examples of individualized education programs, *The Illinois Primer on Individualized Education Programs* presents a step-by-step description of IEP development (State Board of Education et al., 1979). Figure 6-4 illustrates this 18-step process. The reader will note that not all parts of the IEP are required under PL 94-142; some are in compliance with State Rules and Regulations. Although many steps illustrated in Figure 6-4 are self-explanatory, a brief description of each procedure is presented.

Step 1: The date of the multidisciplinary conference and conference participants are recorded. When included on the IEP, the need to prepare a separate report on that conference is eliminated.

Step 2: The conference participants obtain a composite understanding of the child's abilities and disabilities. Placement and IEP development are then based on this profile.

Step 3: The child's current functioning is described. This description

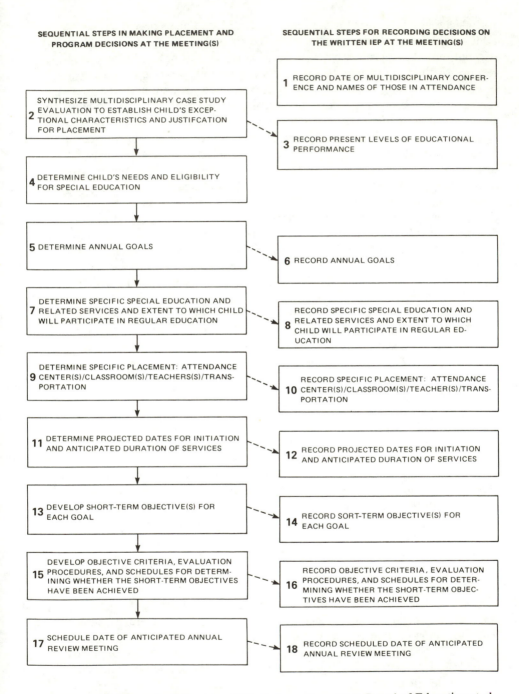

SEQUENTIAL STEPS IN MAKING PLACEMENT AND PROGRAM DECISIONS AT THE MEETING(S)

SEQUENTIAL STEPS FOR RECORDING DECISIONS ON THE WRITTEN IEP AT THE MEETING(S)

1 RECORD DATE OF MULTIDISCIPLINARY CONFERENCE AND NAMES OF THOSE IN ATTENDANCE

2 SYNTHESIZE MULTIDISCIPLINARY CASE STUDY EVALUATION TO ESTABLISH CHILD'S EXCEPTIONAL CHARACTERISTICS AND JUSTIFCATION FOR PLACEMENT

3 RECORD PRESENT LEVELS OF EDUCATIONAL PERFORMANCE

4 DETERMINE CHILD'S NEEDS AND ELIGIBILITY FOR SPECIAL EDUCATION

5 DETERMINE ANNUAL GOALS

6 RECORD ANNUAL GOALS

7 DETERMINE SPECIFIC SPECIAL EDUCATION AND RELATED SERVICES AND EXTENT TO WHICH CHILD WILL PARTICIPATE IN REGULAR EDUCATION

8 RECORD SPECIFIC SPECIAL EDUCATION AND RELATED SERVICES AND EXTENT TO WHICH CHILD WILL PARTICIPATE IN REGULAR EDUCATION

9 DETERMINE SPECIFIC PLACEMENT: ATTENDANCE CENTER(S)/CLASSROOM(S)/TEACHERS(S)/TRANSPORTATION

10 RECORD SPECIFIC PLACEMENT: ATTENDANCE CENTER(S)/CLASSROOM(S)/TEACHER(S)/TRANSPORTATION

11 DETERMINE PROJECTED DATES FOR INITIATION AND ANTICIPATED DURATION OF SERVICES

12 RECORD PROJECTED DATES FOR INITIATION AND ANTICIPATED DURATION OF SERVICES

13 DEVELOP SHORT-TERM OBJECTIVE(S) FOR EACH GOAL

14 RECORD SORT-TERM OBJECTIVE(S) FOR EACH GOAL

15 DEVELOP OBJECTIVE CRITERIA, EVALUATION PROCEDURES, AND SCHEDULES FOR DETERMINING WHETHER THE SHORT-TERM OBJECTIVES HAVE BEEN ACHIEVED

16 RECORD OBJECTIVE CRITERIA, EVALUATION PROCEDURES, AND SCHEDULES FOR DETERMINING WHETHER THE SHORT-TERM OBJECTIVES HAVE BEEN ACHIEVED

17 SCHEDULE DATE OF ANTICIPATED ANNUAL REVIEW MEETING

18 RECORD SCHEDULED DATE OF ANTICIPATED ANNUAL REVIEW MEETING

Figure 6-4. Development of a written IEP. Redrawn from State Board of Education et al., 1979. Courtesy of Illinois Office of Education.

must be based on the results of more than one test and must encompass all areas which might be related to the disability.

Step 4: After the child's strengths and weaknesses have been reviewed, his or her need and eligibility for special services are determined.

Step 5: Once the child's needs are identified, annual goals are established and assigned priorities.

Step 6: The goals developed in Step 5 are recorded on the IEP. It is important that goals relate to the individual child rather than to the child's educational placement.

Step 7: On the basis of the identified needs of the child, appropriate placement and programming are determined. In compliance with the mandates of PL 94-142, the least restrictive, yet appropriate, educational environment is selected. Insofar as possible, the child should be allowed some participation in the regular educational program.

Step 8: The recommendations made in Step 7 are included on the IEP.

Step 9: After the categorical placement for the child and the required support services have been determined, specific placement is made. The following rules and regulations must be considered in making these decisions:

- The placement should be commensurate with the child's needs and should allow for interaction with nonhandicapped children.
- The placement must comply with the specifications of the IEP and should be close to the child's home.
- The child should be educated, if possible, in the school the child would have attended were he or she not in need of special education.
- The effect of the placement on the child and on other children in the selected educational setting must be considered.

The child is assigned to a school, classroom, and teacher after considering the foregoing factors. Transportation arrangements are made if necessary. These arrangements may include a change in the child's mode of transportation, as well as any vehicle adaptation that might be required. It is recommended that travel time to and from school not exceed one hour each way and that this travel not prevent the child from receiving a full day of instruction. The *Illinois Primer* suggests that the IEP meeting might be adjourned after completing Step 9. Convening a second meeting would allow the receiving teacher specified in this step to be involved in the development of short-term objectives.

Step 10: The decisions reached in Step 9 are recorded on the IEP.

Step 11: The dates for initiation of services and an estimate of the duration of such services are determined.

Step 12: The projected dates are included in the IEP.

Step 13: Short-term objectives related to each goal are developed. Each goal must have such objectives.

Step 14: The objectives are included in the IEP.

Step 15: Having established goals and objectives, methods and criteria for measuring progress are established. Target dates for the assessment of short-term objectives are also determined.

Step 16: The criteria, evaluative methods, and projected dates are recorded on the IEP.

Step 17: A date for the annual review is determined.

Step 18: This date is recorded on the IEP.

The Illinois Primer on Individualized Education Programs, then, provides special educators in the state with specific guidelines in IEP development. In addition, districts within the state have generated forms designed to incorporate the required components into a comprehensive document. Figure 6-5 presents one such effort. Similarly, specific guidelines for the content of IEPs are presented in the next section.

IEP CONTENT

According to Illinois and Federal rules and regulations, five components must comprise the IEP. First, the child's present level of functioning must be described. For example, if a child has an articulatory disorder, this statement will include as a minimum the results of formal testing; a description of articulation in conversational speech; and the results of supplementary testing, such as audiometric assessment and examination of the speech mechanisms. The *Illinois Primer* suggests that qualitative, quantitative, and descriptive information be included in this statement.

Second, the *annual goals* and *short-term objectives* must be outlined. Although the former must be somewhat general, a simple statement to the effect that the child will improve his articulatory abilities is inadequate. If several goals are projected, these should be assigned priorities. In the case of short-term objectives, detail is mandatory. The objectives must not only relate to the annual goals but must describe the target behavior, the circumstances under which the behavior should occur, and the criteria to be employed to measure progress. Short-term objectives must not be confused with *session plans;* session plans are based on the objectives, just as the objectives are based on the annual goals. As the *Illinois Primer* suggests, "a short-term instructional objective specifies a culminating behavior resulting from a series of instructional activities" (State Board of Education et al., 1979). These instructional activities are included in daily session plans. Table 6-1 illustrates the relationship between annual goals, short-term objectives, and instructional activities.

The third required component of an IEP is specification of the educational and related services to be provided to the child and a statement regarding the extent to which the child can function in regular educational programs.

EAST DUPAGE SPECIAL EDUCATION DISTRICT (Districts 4, 45, 48, 88 and 205)

502 E. Van Buren   Villa Park, IL   60181   279-4725

☐ Multidisciplinary Conference   Conference Date:_____
☐ Individual Education Program   ☐ New ☐ Continuing ☐ Change ☐ Transfer ☐ Termination
☐ Annual Review

Student Name:_____   Birthdate:_____ CA:_____ ID#_____
Address:_____   Phone:_____ District:_____
                                          Home School:_____
Parents/Guardian:_____   Ethnic Background:_____
Address (if different):_____   Language (student):_____

Exceptional Characteristics:	Primary	Secondary
A Trainable Mentally Handicapped	☐	☐
B Educable Mentally Handicapped	☐	☐
C Physically Handicapped	☐	☐
D Learning Disabled	☐	☐
E Visually Impaired	☐	☐
F Hard-of-Hearing	☐	☐
G Deaf	☐	☐
H Deaf/Blind	☐	☐
I Speech/Language Impaired	☐	☐
J Educationally Handicapped	☐	☐
K Behavior Disorder	☐	☐
L Other Health	☐	☐
M Multiply Handicapped	☐	☐

Standard Education Placement: District_____ Grade_____
Teacher_____ School_____
☐ Private ☐ Public ☐ Parochial

Special Education Placement:
☐ District Prog.   ☐ Joint Agreement Prog.   ☐ DuPage/West
☐ Related Services   Cook Regional
☐ Resource Program (less than 50%)
☐ Instructional Program (50% or more) estimate %_____
☐ Nonpublic   ☐ Residential
☐ Preschool ☐ Full Day   ☐ Half Day
Teacher_____ # Aide_____ # Pupils_____
Program_____   LRE_____
District #_____ School_____
Projected Starting Date_____
Projected Review_____ Re-eval. Date_____

☐ 14-7.02   ☐ 14-7.02a   ☐ 14-7.03

PARTICIPANTS

Special Education Director (Designee)_____   Teacher(s)_____
Princial (Designee)_____   _____
                                                       _____
Joint Agreement Personnel_____   _____
_____   Social Worker_____
_____   Speech/Language Pathologist____
_____   Nurse_____
                                                       Counselor_____
Parent(s)/Guardian_____   Other (Specify Title)_____
Student_____   _____
Psychologist_____   _____

Purpose of Staffing_____
Justification for Placement_____

Recommendations:_____
_____
_____

Transportation: ☐ Yes   ☐ No

Yes	No	
		The following were explained: ☐ Multidisciplinary Staff Conference ☐ Recommended Placement ☐ Individual Education Program
___	___	I/We request a copy of my child's educational program and understand within 30 days short term instructional objectives will be completed.
___	___	I/We agree with and understand the recommendations concerning placement.
___	___	I/We agree to waive the ten (10) school day preplacement period.
___	___	I/We agree with the proposed evaluation(s).
		Legal rights, including the right to object to placement, were explained and offered in writing, if requested.

Date:_____
        Signature: Parents or Guardian   Staff Member Preparing Conference Report

☐ Parent(s) not in attendance   ☐ Parent(s) to be notified by mail/phone   Notified By:_____ Date:_____

cc: District/White   Parent/Yellow   Teacher/Pink   EDSED/Gold   10-79

Figure 6-5. East Dupage Special Education District IEP form. Courtesy of Public Schools District 45, Villa Park, Illinois.

Table 6-1
Instructional Objectives for Mathematics
Annual Goal: Student will learn multiplication and division computation skills

Short-Term Objective	Evaluation of Short-Term Objectives				Results of Evaluation Skills		
	Tests, Materials, Evaluation Procedures	Criteria of Successful Performance	Evaluation Schedule	Date Objective Mastered	Not Existing	Emerging	Acquired
Student will add numbers involving two renamings	Computation of 20 addition problems requiring two re-namings	85% accuracy	End of first grading period	10/10/79			X
Student will subtract numbers involving two renamings	Computation of 20 subtraction problems requiring two re-namings	85% accuracy	End of second grading period	11/14/79			X
Student will multiply and divide through products of 81	Completion of fact sheet containing 20 multiplication and division facts, and products through 81 within a specified time	65% accuracy	End of third grading period	1/15/80		X	
Student will multiply two digit numbers by one digit numbers	Completion of appropriate mastery test in mathematics text	75% accuracy	End of fourth grading period			X	
Student will divide numbers by two digit divisors	Completion of appropriate mastery test in mathematics text	75% accuracy	End of fifth grading period				

SOURCE: Based on State Board of Education et al., 1979. Courtesy of Illinois Office of Education.

If the child is disordered only in the area of communication, a statement regarding the most appropriate service delivery option is required. Would the child benefit from supportive services from the school speech-language pathologist, or is placement in a language classroom or resource room necessary? If such placement is required, what percentage of the school day, if any, can the child spend in the regular classroom or interacting with non-handicapped children? Placement must be in the classroom closest to the child's home, and transportation may need to be arranged.

The fourth requirement is an estimate of the duration of services and the projected date for their initiation. When the child requires multiple services, differing duration dates may be projected. None should exceed one year, however. The fifth requirement is specification of the evaluative procedures and criteria. These assessments, to be made on at least an annual basis, determine whether the objectives are being reached.

In addition to the five items specified by law, the *Illinois Primer* suggests "best practice components," which include the following:

- Date of multidisciplinary conference and names of the participants
- Statement of long range goals
- Name of person or persons responsible for implementing the goals and objectives
- Specification of special instructional media and materials
- Space for noting the child's strengths and talents
- Names of participants in attendance at the IEP meeting
- Parents' rights checklist

All states have undoubtedly prepared guidelines for developing both IEPs and the forms to be employed, and it was simply ready access to Illinois materials that led to their inclusion in this chapter. Some forms are specific (Fig. 6-6), whereas others tend to be general in nature (Fig. 6-7). The reader is encouraged to seek additional IEP specimens from local school speech-language pathologists, and to refer to Dublinske (1978) for further information on IEP development.

ISSUES SURROUNDING IEPs

Since IEPs became mandatory, many issues regarding their development and implementation have surfaced. The National Association of State Directors of Special Education (undated), for example, published a *Summary of research findings on individualized education programs.* The first project, entitled the "Connecticut Study," dealt with the participation of team members in the IEP process. A total of 1478 persons involved in 230 Planning Teams (PT) were surveyed. The researchers were specifically interested in the levels

NAME: _____ I.D.: _____ SESSIONS PER WEEK: _____ YEAR: _____
D.O.B.: _____ AGE: _____ GRADE: _____ SCHOOL: _____ FACILITATOR: _____
PARTICIPANTS IN DEVELOPMENT OF I.E.P.: _____
PRESENT STATUS: _____

	DATE BEGAN	OBJ. REACHED YES NO	DATE

1. GOAL: Acquire auditory skills related to production of _____.
   OBJECTIVES
   A. Recognize _____ in isolation with _____ % accuracy in _____ trials.
   B. Recognize _____ in words with _____ % accuracy in _____ trials.
   C. Discriminate correct and incorrect _____ with _____ % accuracy in _____ trials.

2. GOAL: Produce _____ in isolation.
   OBJECTIVES
   A. Use correct placement of articulators for _____ with _____ % accuracy in _____ trials.
   B. Produce _____ in isolation with _____ % accuracy in _____ trials.

3. GOAL: Produce _____ in syllables.
   OBJECTIVES
   A. Produce _____ in consonant-vowel combination with _____ % accuracy in _____ trials.
   B. Produce _____ in vowel-consonant with _____ % accuracy in _____ trials.
   C. Produce _____ in consonant-vowel-consonent with _____ % accuracy in _____ trials.

4. GOAL: Produce _____ in words.
   OBJECTIVES
   A. Produce _____ in initial position of words with _____ % accuracy in _____ trials.
   B. Produce _____ in final position of words with _____ % accuracy in _____ trials.
   C. Produce _____ in medial position of words with _____ % accuracy in _____ trials.
   D. Produce _____ in blends with _____ % accuracy in _____ trials.

5. GOAL: Use of _____ in structured speech situations.
   OBJECTIVES
   A. Use _____ in sentences with _____ % accuracy in _____ trials.
   B. Use _____ in oral reading with _____ % accuracy in _____ trials.
   C. Use _____ in controlled conversation with _____ % accuracy in _____ trials.
   D. Other: _____

6. GOAL: Establish carryover of _____.
   OBJECTIVES
   A. Use _____ with _____ % accuracy in _____ therapy sessions.
   B. Use _____ with _____ % accuracy when observed in the classroom.
   C. Other: _____

SUMMARY AND RECOMMENDATIONS: _____

D.O.C.: w/Master File, y/Sp.P., p/Parent, g/Parent   ANNUAL REVIEW DATE: _____   PARENTS DID / DID NOT ATTEND
REV.: 05-80

Figure 6-6. Peoria Public Schools, District 150, Special Services Division, Form S/L #6: Individual Educational Program—Articulation. Courtesy of Peoria Public Schools.

NAME: _____ AGE: _____ GRADE: _____ I.D.#: _____ SESSIONS PER WEEK: _____ YEAR: _____
D.O.B.: _____
PARTICIPANTS IN DEVELOPMENT OF I.E.P.: _____ SCHOOL: _____ FACILITATOR: _____
PRESENT STATUS: _____
LANGUAGE AREAS: Concepts, Vocabulary, Syntax, Auditory Memory, Auditory Discrimination, Auditory Processing, Association.
                 Categorization, Sequencing, Mean Length of Response, Other.

			DATE BEGAN	OBJ. REACHED YES NO	DATE

1. GOAL: _____

   OBJECTIVES
   A. _____ with _____ % accuracy in _____ trials.   ___ ___ ___ ___
   B. _____ with _____ % accuracy in _____ trials.   ___ ___ ___ ___
   C. _____ with _____ % accuracy in _____ trials.   ___ ___ ___ ___

2. GOAL: _____

   OBJECTIVES
   A. _____ with _____ % accuracy in _____ trials.   ___ ___ ___ ___
   B. _____ with _____ % accuracy in _____ trials.   ___ ___ ___ ___
   C. _____ with _____ % accuracy in _____ trials.   ___ ___ ___ ___

3. GOAL: _____

   OBJECTIVES
   A. _____ with _____ % accuracy in _____ trials.   ___ ___ ___ ___
   B. _____ with _____ % accuracy in _____ trials.   ___ ___ ___ ___
   C. _____ with _____ % accuracy in _____ trials.   ___ ___ ___ ___

4. GOAL: _____

   OBJECTIVES
   A. _____ with _____ % accuracy in _____ trials.   ___ ___ ___ ___
   B. _____ with _____ % accuracy in _____ trials.   ___ ___ ___ ___
   C. _____ with _____ % accuracy in _____ trials.   ___ ___ ___ ___

5. GOAL: _____

   OBJECTIVES
   A. _____ with _____ % accuracy in _____ trials.   ___ ___ ___ ___
   B. _____ with _____ % accuracy in _____ trials.   ___ ___ ___ ___
   C. _____ with _____ % accuracy in _____ trials.   ___ ___ ___ ___

SUMMARY AND RECOMMENDATIONS: _____

D.O.C.: w/Master File, y/Sp.P., p/Parent, g/Parent   ANNUAL REVIEW DATE: _____   PARENTS DID / DID NOT ATTEND
REV.: 05-80

Figure 6-7. Peoria Public Schools, District 150, Special Services Division, Form S/L #7: Individual Educational Program—Language. Courtesy of Peoria Public Schools.

of participation and satisfaction of PT members, PT members' understanding of their roles, and their decision-making styles, as well as the roles played by parents in the IEP process.

Among the findings of the survey was that because communication was oral rather than written, it was sometimes inadequate. The researchers also found that Planning Team conferences were usually dominated by administrators and appraisal personnel, while teachers played rather passive roles. This was attributed to the presence of building principals at the meetings. Because personal satisfaction seemed to be directly related to degree of participation, teachers were disenchanted with the conferences. With regard to role understanding, the participants were not cognizant of the purposes and scope of committee activities, and teachers seemed to be the least well informed. Moreover, the researchers found that decisions were being made by one or two PT members rather than by the entire group. Finally, the parents' role in planning was not well defined. Although they provided information to the PT, parents were not expected to participate in decision making.

James D. Marver and Jane L. David analyzed 150 IEPs and interviewed 200 parents, teachers, and administrators between October 1976 and September 1977 (National Association of State Directors of Special Education, undated). Regarding preplacement preparation, the researchers found that early parent notification was beneficial but that parents were not included in the preplanning meetings. Assessment of children with potential problems was inefficient. Frequently, examiners were not trained, the process was incomplete, and assessment guidelines were not available. The researchers found that at IEP meetings, committee size ranged from 3 to 15 members. They also found that because meetings were held before or after school, or at noon, the teachers' unions were displeased. Although parents participated in 60 to 90 percent of the cases, their contribution in meetings was inconsequential. Child participation was found to be nonexistent.

Marver and David's review of IEPs revealed that emphasis was on special education, rather than special and regular educational programming. Although compliance with state IEP regulations was apparent, the quality of IEPs differed from district to district. Confusion between goals and objectives was revealed, and staff members agreed that they needed training in the IEP process and development. Finally, even though the staff were aware that the IEP was not legally binding, they seemed to be fearful of their accountability as it related to IEP content. With regard to placement, the researchers found that the time span from identification to placement ranged from two weeks to six months; six weeks was the average. On a positive note, the researchers reported that handicapped children were being identified more frequently and that the services provided to these children were improving.

Among the issues studied by Pat Morrissey and Nancy Hafer was the parental role in the IEP process (National Association of State Directors of

Special Education, undated). The researchers interviewd 1000 persons in four states, including representatives of state education agencies, school personnel, parents of exceptional children, and members of advocacy groups. Both parents and school personnel expressed concern about parents' capacity for participation in the IEP process. Representatives from the schools felt that parents were unprepared to participate in educational program development. Although parents concurred with this reservation, they did feel that they could provide useful information to the planning team and should participate in the IEP review.

Some concern related to the costs of parental participation when compared to the benefits derived from such involvement. It was noted that conferences were sometimes held after school or in the evenings, and home visits were occasionally necessary to obtain parental consent. Formal notification and consent procedures resulted in some delays in initiating services.

The role of the teacher in the IEP process was also explored. Teachers expressed concern about the time consumed by noninstructional activities and by activities for which they were not trained. The teachers further appeared to view the IEP mandate of PL 94-142 as "an expression of lack of faith in the ability of out nation's teachers to effectively educate handicapped children (National Association of State Directors of Special Education, undated, p. 12).

There were positive reports from the teachers. Many considered the IEP process helpful in their teaching. The methods of measuring progress not only assisted the teachers but also served to motivate and involve students. In general, however, the teachers felt that they needed additional training in order to execute their responsibilities in the IEP process effectively.

The importance of seeking assistance from allied professionals and working with the parents of nonhandicapped children was stressed by Reynolds (1978). He suggested that special educators could learn from sociologists about family interactions and that psychologists could help educators develop clinical skills for IEP conferences. For example, in order to function adequately in IEP meetings, educators must learn to listen to parents, must be willing to share in decision making, and must improve their ability to share different perspectives about children with others. Reynolds also indicated that special educators were obligated to inform parents of nonhandicapped children about PL 94-142 and the impact of that legislation on their children. The latter children must be taught to deal with the handicapped children in their classrooms, and it is the teacher's responsibility to create a supportive and cooperative social environment within that room. In short, Reynolds states that the IEP process should be a cooperative, sharing effort among professionals, parents, and children.

REFERENCES

Dublinske, S. P.L. 94-142: Developing the individualized education program (IEP). *Asha*, 1978, *20*, 380–397.

National Association of State Directors of Special Education. *Summary of research findings on individualized education programs*. Undated.

North Dakota Department of Public Instruction. *Special education in North Dakota guidelines III: Programs for students with language, speech and hearing disorders in the public schools*. 1977.

Public Law 94-142, *Education for All Handicapped Children Act of 1975*.

Reynolds, M. C. Staying out of jail. *Teaching Exceptional Children*, 1978, *10*, 60–62.

State Board of Education, Illinois Office of Education, Department of Specialized Educational Services, and Illinois Regional Resource Center. *The Illinois primer on individualized education programs*. Springfield, Illinois, June 1979.

7

Service Delivery

Every child has a need to develop maximum competence in communica-
tion—listening, speaking, reading, and writing—and school programs
have a continuing responsibility to meet the communicative needs of all
children and youth. (American Speech and Hearing Association,
1973-1974)

In 1965, if one were asked to visualize the school "speech therapist" in his or
her natural habitat, one might conjure up a picture of a professional working
in cramped quarters in an elementary school and at a small table with three or
four lisping youngsters. Today, in 1981, the basic scene might be the same,
but it is probable that the speech-language pathologist is modifying techniques and moving into other settings in order to meet the needs of previously
unserved or underserved children and adolescents. Among the children
unserved by the school speech-language pathologist in the past were preschoolers; because students are now exposed to this age group and trained to
work with them, the delivery of services to these youngsters should not present problems. Most preprofessional and graduate students also have had experiences with children presenting multiple disorders. It is questionable,
however, whether the training and experiences currently provided prepare
professionals to work with culturally different children. Similarly, experience
suggests that exposure to adolescents may be limited, and it is almost certain
that few students have had the opportunity to work with incarcerated
adolescents. These groups of students may all be classified as underserved in
the school setting.

PHYSICAL FACILITIES AND EQUIPMENT

The physical setting in which speech-language pathologists function has received a great deal of attention in teachers' rooms; in local, state, and national meetings; and in other forums in which schools speech-language pathologists congregate. Inadequate rooms that are inappropriately located and equipped have frequently been described and discussed by school personnel in informal conversation. Less frequent attention has been accorded "speech rooms" in the professional literature. In the following discussion, recommendations for the housing of school speech-language programs are presented; consideration is also given to the realities of the current status of speech-language pathology facilities in schools.

Luper and Ainsworth (1955) have described speech correction rooms in the school setting. Assuming that larger school systems would include a speech correctionist and a hearing conservation specialist, the authors described a suite designed to accommodate both. The authors pointed out that even in the absence of the latter specialist, the speech correctionist would require these facilities in order to work with hearing impaired children. In one option, a 19' × 10' soundproofed room was designated for audiometric testing and recording. Adjacent to that area was a 21' × 12' combination office and therapy room. Cupboards and a padded bench were built into this room. The bench was to be used as a relaxation table when working with children who stuttered or had cerebral palsy. Cupboards allowed for equipment and material storage. Numerous wall receptables were planned to permit the utilization of equipment without inconvenience.

In an alternate plan, a 22' × 20' soundproofed room was proposed. It, too, had 30" high cupboards, a padded bench, and numerous electrical outlets. The authors emphasized that both rooms should be well lighted and ventilated, should contain adequate storage space, and should have a blackboard, bulletin board, and mounted mirror. Although furnishings and equipment were not specified, it was suggested that a low table and chairs of various sizes were imperative.

Despite the optimism expressed by Luper and Ainsworth that the necessity of adequate facilities for school speech-language pathologists would be acknowledged by school districts, a survey several years later indicated that their optimism was premature (Knight, Hahn, Ervin, & McIssac, 1961). A total of 705 speech-language pathologists across the country were asked to rate their physical facilities, equipment, materials, and supplies as "excellent," "adequate," or "wanting." Only 12 percent of the respondents indicated that their therapy rooms were "excellent," and 50 percent reported that their physical facilities were "wanting." Greater satisfaction was expressed regarding equipment, materials, and supplies. Only 31 percent of respondents indicated that their equipment was "wanting"; 21 percent and

18 percent felt their materials and supplies, respectively, were inadequate. Approximately 50 percent of respondents felt their needs in these areas were being adequately met. Respondents frequently noted that, because no room was specified for their utilization, it was necessary to transport materials and equipment from school to school. In general, the surveyed speech-language pathologists were not satisfied with their physical accommodations but were less unhappy about equipment, materials, and supplies available for their use.

Addressing the subjects of speech rooms and therapy equipment, Black acknowledged that ideal situations are rarely encountered. Nevertheless, she made recommendations regarding the design, location, and equipping of functional therapy areas. The speech room should be located in a relatively quiet area of the school, close to the primary classrooms. Although the speech-language pathologist is frequently asked to share space with other professionals or programs, Black emphasized that certain areas should be avoided; these include the health room and the teacher's room.

The speech room should be large enough to accommodate eight students. The itinerant speech-language pathologist should also have an office in one of the buildings. This office should contain a desk, phone, filing cabinet, and storage area. In a larger therapy room, the office area could be partitioned off from the therapy space. According to Black, the therapy room should be sound-treated to permit reliable audiometric testing and the preparation of tape recordings. Further, the room should be well lighted, well ventilated, and attractively decorated.

Black differentiated between the spatial needs for elementary and secondary school programs. For the most part, younger students attend therapy for a designated period and then return to their classrooms. However, it is sometimes necessary to schedule high school pupils for 60-minute periods. During this time, the speech-language pathologist may choose to work directly with students for 20–30 minutes and then to allow them to practice independently for the remainder of the hour. If, during this practice period, the speech-language pathologist wishes to provide direct services to other students, practice cubicles or areas for the students are needed. Figure 7-1 illustrates a therapy room appropriate for an elementary school, and Figure 7-2 represents well-designed high school accommodations.

Black specified basic equipment needs for a speech room. Included were tables and chairs appropriate for small children as well as older students; two tables (of different dimensions) were recommended (see Figure 7-1) in order to accommodate the physical differences between kindergartners and sixth grade students. Adult chairs should be provided for the speech-language pathologist, parents, and/or visitors. Black also recommended that the speech-language pathologist's office contain a teacher's desk, typewriter, and file cabinet. And, according to Black (1964), "a therapist with Freudian or Edna Hill Young orientation may want a cot for therapy, or she may need it

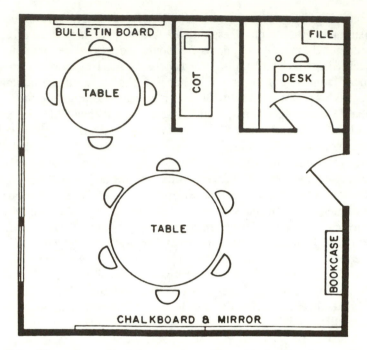

Figure 7-1. Elementary school therapy room. From Black, *Speech correction in the schools,* © 1964, pp. 42–44. Reprinted by permission of Prentice-Hall, Inc., Englewood Cliffs, New Jersey.

for her own differential relaxation after the last small child lisps his way back to the classroom'' (pp. 44–45). Storage areas, a mirror, and a bulletin board were also considered part of the basic equipment needs of an adequate therapy room. Among the instructional materials recommended were tape recorders, auditory trainers, musical instruments, record players, visual aids, games, and audiometers.

In a report published in *Asha,* the American Speech and Hearing Association (ASHA) Subcommittee on Housing of the Committee on Speech and Hearing Services in the Schools (1969) recognized that the adequacy of physical setting and equipment influenced the effectiveness of therapy programs and made recommendations regarding speech rooms, furniture, storage facilities, and equipment. The speech room, in addition to being located in a quiet area of the building, was to be situated near the administrative unit and accessible to the classrooms, the school secretary, the waiting area, and the offices of other other special service personnel. With a recommended size of 150–250 square feet, the speech room should have both artificial and natural lighting and, ideally, should have an adjacent office. Minimally, the room should be accoustically treated; drapes and carpeting

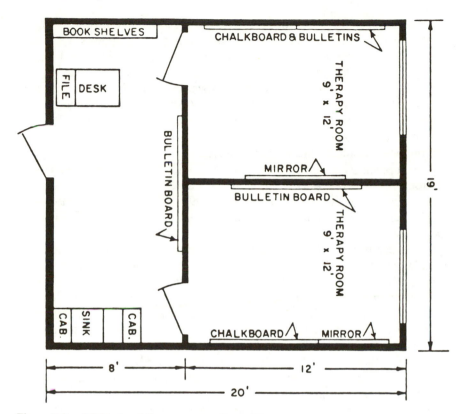

Figure 7-2. High school therapy room. From Black, *Speech correction in the schools,* © 1964, pp. 42–44. Reprinted by permission of Prentice-Hall, Inc., Englewood Cliffs, New Jersey.

are considered ideal. An intercom system connected to the administrative unit was also regarded as ideal. The Subcommittee specified that the room should have at least one electrical outlet, and that a chalkboard, bulletin board, and mirror—each approximately 3′ × 5′ in size—should be mounted on the walls.

With regard to furniture, an office desk, at least two adult chairs, an adjustable table, a variety of childrens' chairs, and an equipment stand were recommended. Storage facilities included a locked file cabinet, locked storage space, and a book case. Finally, equipment needs were specified. An audiometer, auditory training equipment, and a tape recorder were recommended. Additionally, the speech-language pathologist should have access to a phonograph and a typewriter. A telephone (preferably with a direct line), an electric clock, and a wastebasket should also be present in the therapy room.

The Professional Services Board (PSB) of ASHA has published guidelines for school programs for communicatively disordered children (American Speech and Hearing Association, 1973–1974). In discussing the

physical plant and equipment needed to provide effective professional services, the PSB recommended that the facility be private, quiet, and of adequate size. The therapy areas should be accessible to physically handicapped
children (when relevant); all newly constructed rooms should be barrier-free.
Adequate lighting and ventilation were specified, and the Board indicated
that several electrical outlets should be present in the facility. Storage space, a
locked file, and appropriately sized tables and chairs should be provided. The
report indicated that mobile units or prefabricated buildings should be considered when available facilities are inadequate.

Equipment needs identified by the Professional Services Board included
audiometers, tape recorders, and auditory trainers. Diagnostic tools and instructional materials were also specified. When special populations are to
receive services, additional equipment and architectural adaptations may be
necessary.

Alluded to in the PSB Standards and Guidelines was the utilization of a
mobile speech unit. Howerton (1973) has described the utilization of such
units in Columbia County, Florida. Unable to locate appropriate facilities in
the overcrowded public schools, the author investigated the availability and
relative cost of mobile units. Howerton found that it was less expensive to
build and equip a mobile classroom than to provide appropriate facilities in
the schools serviced by the unit.

The author reported satisfaction with the mobile speech unit. He indicated that the children enjoyed leaving the building in order to attend
speech sessions. An important advantage in utilizing a mobile unit is that all
equipment, materials, and records are in a single location. Howerton said
that he made better use of various pieces of equipment in the mobile unit than
he did when transportation of this equipment was necessary. In short, the
author indicated that a properly equipped and located mobile speech unit was
economical, as well as conducive to the provision of effective therapeutic services. Figures 7-3 and 7-4 illustrate two mobile units designed for use by
speech-language pathologists.

Although this may be the exception rather than the rule, at least one state
describes the facilities that should be provided for school speech, language,
and hearing programs. North Dakota guidelines state that "There shall be an
established quiet place appropriate to program and student needs. Storage for
equipment and materials and adequate light, heat, and ventilation are also required" (North Dakota Department of Public Instruction, 1977, p. 6).

The speech room, according to North Dakota regulations, should be
near classrooms and free from health and safety hazards. The minimal size of
the facility should be 180 square feet, and two electrical outlets should be provided. There should also be access to the building's intercommunication
system. The facility should contain an office chair and desk, appropriately
sized table and chairs, and a filing cabinet. A bulletin board, blackboard, and

mirror should also be present in the room. Finally, a tape recorder, an audiometer, and funds to purchase therapy materials must be provided to the speech-language pathologist. Part-time clerical help should also be available.

These, then, are some of the recommendations made regarding the physical facilities in which school speech-language pathologists should function. Equipment and miscellaneous materials have also been specified by some of the recommending agencies. Although undoubtedly many public school facilities meet the standards outlined in the previous discussion, an equal number may not. The following illustrations emphasize this point.

When the author was a public school speech-language pathologist in the early 1960s, her assigned speech rooms were clearly inadequate. In one building, the speech room was located adjacent to the patrol boy's equipment storage area. In fact, access to the room was through this storage area. The 8' × 10' room contained an adult-size table, four large chairs, and one movable locked storage unit. A reversible blackboard-mirror unit was also provided. One light located on a high ceiling provided inadequate lighting, but this was compensated for (on sunny days) by natural light coming through a single window. The room was relatively quiet, since it was located on the second floor of the building and well removed from the noisy primary classrooms. This serene environment was disrupted at the beginning of the school day and at lunch time, however, when the patrol boys collected their equipment. Figure 7-5 represents the speech room in School A.

As is apparent from the diagram, the room was inadequately equipped. The audiometer, auditory trainers, and tape recorders recommended by various agencies were not provided. Only a screening test of articulation was available, along with a variety of partially complete commercial games. The school did not furnish any supplies, although limited materials were available through the special education office.

In School B, the equipment, supplies, and therapy materials were no better but the physical facilities were new and cheerful. Located in a recently constructed building, the speech room was well lighted and well ventilated. Two large mounted blackboards, along with a small table and chairs, an office desk and chair, the usual movable storage unit, and reversible mirror-blackboard were provided. Unfortunately, the speech room also served as the health and teacher preparation room. A duplicating machine, sink, and first aid cabinet were also in the speech room and teachers sometimes disrupted therapy by duplicating materials during sessions. Injured students also appeared frequently to have their wounds bandaged, their temperatures taken, and their major and minor illnesses diagnosed. Since the school nurse was not in the building daily, the author foolishly attended to some of the less serious physical problems at the expense of therapy time (and also at the risk of a malpractice suit). Figure 7-6 illustrates this multipurpose room in School B.

In the other three schools services by the author over a five-year period,

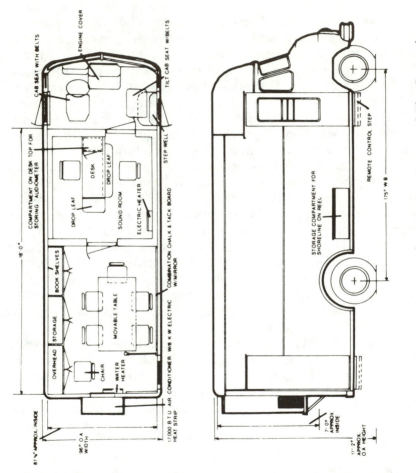
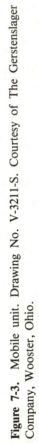

Figure 7-3. Mobile unit. Drawing No. V-3211-S. Courtesy of The Gerstenslager Company, Wooster, Ohio.

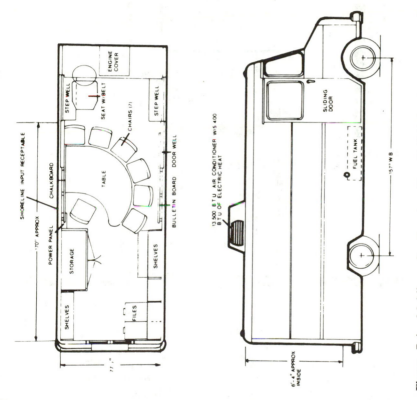

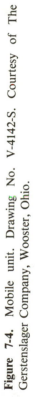

Figure 7-4. Mobile unit. Drawing No. V-4142-S. Courtesy of The Gerstenslager Company, Wooster, Ohio.

117

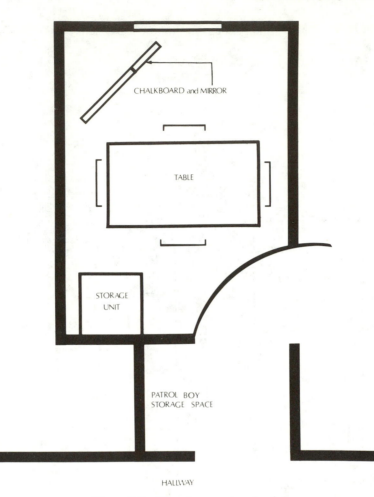

Figure 7-5. Speech room in school A.

the situations were not appreciably better. One room doubled as the art supply room; needless to say, this was a helpful source of tagboard, colored paper, and other therapy-related materials. (All acquisitions, of course, were made with the knowledge of the building principal!) Another room was rather large and, when properly decorated, it evolved into a rather comfortable facility. Unfortunately, it was *too* large, *too* attractive, and *too* comfortable; thus it was quickly transformed into a resource area for the entire school. The fifth speech room was also large; it accommodated two office desks and chairs, a children's table and chairs, the movable storage unit, and the reversible blackboard and mirror combination quite nicely. Two mounted blackboards and a bulletin board covered three walls, and windows occupied

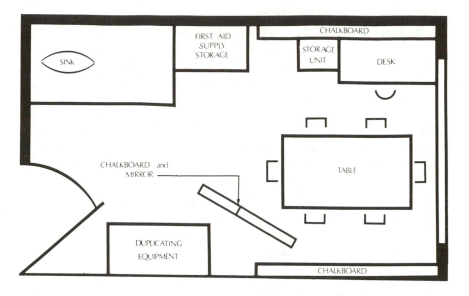

Figure 7-6. Multipurpose (speech, health, and teacher-preparation) room in School B.

the other wall. Although the artifical illumination was inadequate, natural lighting compensated to a great extent. The major problem here was the room's location within the building. This school, which accommodated approximately 1000 students, had three distinctive sections. The speech room was located in the oldest section of the building, on an upward extension of the second floor. An addition connected the original building to the most recently constructed primary wing. The reader will understand why so many young children arrived late for therapy or missed sessions altogether as a result of "losing their way."

The passage of 15 years has not produced a noticeable improvement in the conditions under which school speech-language pathologists work. In the past few years, the author has supervised students working under certified school speech-language pathologists in teachers' rooms, furnace rooms, and "coat closets." Speech rooms were also located adjacent to lavatories, music rooms, and gymnasiums. Flushing toilets, off-key musicians, and yelling athletes do not provide suitable acoustic environments for perfecting articulatory, linguistic, fluency, or vocal skills. The overwhelming majority of speech rooms had architectural barriers that would preclude the servicing of nonambulatory children. In fact, at least one room was so small that the student clinician could not be supervised unless the supervisor sat outside in the hall. Recently an experienced school speech-language pathologist confided to the author that her current speech room has only a table and chairs and that she keeps her session plans and IEPs in a cardboard box!

With declining school enrollments and increasing emphasis on the provision of quality services to speech and language disordered children, it is anticipated that physical accommodations for school speech-language pathologists will improve. It behooves professionals to be aware of recommended standards for such facilities and to seek suitable space and equipment.

It has often been noted that adequate facilities and equipment do not guarantee adequate clinical care; this is particularly true when the speech-language pathologist lacks the background to deal effectively with specific groups of individuals, such as culturally different youths and adolescents.

SERVICE DELIVERY
TO CULTURALLY DIFFERENT CHILDREN

Philosophical Issues and Goal Setting

Perhaps the most difficult part of the speech-language pathologist's role in dealing with culturally different children and adolescents is determining appropriate goals for the therapeutic process. Some believe that all children should use communicative patterns consistent with general American English, and that these patterns should be utilized at all times. The basis of this philosophy is that opportunities for educational, vocational, and social success are dependent on the individual's ability to conform to standard speech and language usage. Others take the somewhat different position that children and young adults should be made aware of the differences between their own communicative patterns and those considered to be standard and that these young people should be encouraged to develop facility in using the latter. On this view, the decision as to whether to employ the original or the acquired linguistic style is situationally dictated. Advocates of this position recognize that the individual may be judged in terms of his or her ability to communicate well with a variety of people in a variety of situations and that shifting of styles will permit such meaningful interaction. At the same time, theoretically, the individual is able to retain the distinctive cultural aspects of his or her language or dialect.

Finally, there is a group of practitioners who feel that it is inappropriate for the speech-language pathologist to impose standard English upon speakers of other languages or dialects. According to these persons, dialect (language) reflects cultural heritage, and modification of these language patterns would dilute or negate the individuality of these groups. The speech-language pathologist with this philosophy might be concerned with substandard variations within individual language-dialectal patterns but would not establish the acquisition of standard English speech and language as a goal.

The decision as to which philosophy to follow is not always an individual one. Some districts have established policies that must be followed in dealing with children whose language reflects cultural differences. It behooves the school speech-language pathologist to determine if such regulations exist in the district prior to implementing programs designed to modify culturally based language differences. This does not imply that individual philosophies based on a sound consideration of the literature should not be developed by the speech-language pathologist; it suggests, rather, that if the policy of the district is not consistent with current thinking and concrete evidence, the speech-language pathologist should be prepared to present convincing information that demonstrates the need for a policy change.

Service Delivery to Speakers of Black English

Bountress (1980) attempted to determine how speech-language pathologists viewed children who speak black English with specific reference to the establishment of therapy goals. Questionnaires were sent to 103 speech-language pathologists working in the school districts of southeastern Virginia. The speech-language pathologists were asked the same questions considered in the preceding discussion. Should speakers of black English learn and employ standard English consistently? Should standard English be taught but black English accepted? Or, should black English be accepted unconditionally? The respondents were also asked to describe their knowledge of black English, as well as to provide some information. Finally, the speech-language pathologists were to indicate whether they felt they needed additional course work in social dialects.

The questionnaire was returned by 100 speech-language pathologists, 21 of whom were black. The mean age of the group was 29, and their professional experience ranged from less than 5 years to more than 15. Of the rspondents, 42 held master's degrees; the remaining 58 held bachelor's degrees. Bountress found that 97 of the 100 respondents taught standard English to speakers of black dialect but allowed those children to retain the nonstandard dialect. Three respondents felt that standard English should be used at all times; not one speech-language pathologist favored the unconditional retention of black English.

The respondents reported that their knowledge of black English was gained from a variety of informational sources: 34 percent obtained such information through course work; 80 percent reported that their knowledge came with experience; and 29 percent of the respondents had attended inservice workshops. As the figures demonstrate, the speech-language pathologists did not rely on a single source for their information. Of the 58 bachelor's-level professionals, over 68 percent felt that they wanted additional course work in the area of social dialects; 66.7 percent of the master's-level speech-language pathogists concurred.

The results of this investigation suggest that speech-language pathologists in Virginia are somewhat united in their philosophies regarding goal-setting for speakers of black English. Because this study was done on a regional basis, the investigator suggests that a national survey be conducted to ascertain if speech-language pathologists across the country concur with this philosophy.

Regardless of speech-language pathologists' goal orientations, they are obligated to evaluate children from differing cultures, and accurate assessment is important. Too frequently, speech-language pathologists have access to a limited number of diagnostic tools, and these may have been standardized on populations quite dissimilar to the target group. The widely used Peabody Picture Vocabulary Test, for example, was normed on a group of white children in Tennessee; is this an appropriate tool to use with black children in Chicago, Illinois? Several adaptations of tests have been made so that Spanish-speaking children may be evaluated, but it is probably safe to assume that many tests currently available to school speech-language pathologists are not always appropriate to the group being tested or sensitive to their specific abilities and disabilities. Therefore, the speech-language pathologist must be cautious in test selection as well as in interpretation of the results.

The materials and procedures to be utilized in working with culturally different children will be influenced by the speech-language pathologist's philosophy of treatment goals. Regardless of philosophic orientation, the appropriate place to begin therapy is with materials and procedures within the experiential realm of the child. The speech-language pathologist who wishes to expand and broaden the child's cultural boundaries can then move into areas somewhat foreign to the child. Emphasis can not be so much on what children have experienced or are experiencing in their neighborhoods or communities, but on what might be encountered if they expand their horizons and increase their abilities. The speech-language pathologist who begins to work with a language disordered inner city child on a unit about farm animals will probably be less effective in providing meaningful experiences than a specialist who begins with something within the child's entry experiences and then moves into other areas. In general, the therapeutic approach, regardless of the perceived communicative disorder, should move from the familiar to the unique; the specific direction of this movement depends on the philosophy of the speech-language pathologist.

For those speech-language pathologists working with culturally disadvantaged children—specifically the inner-city child—Jones (1972) has discussed attributes necessary for successful intervention. First, the speech-language pathologist must know the child. The following are some observations that have been made of disadvantaged, inner-city children:

- Family income is often below subsistence level; educational and vocational achievement are also low among family members.
- More than half of disadvantaged children are from broken homes.

- Untreated medical and dental problems are not uncommon among inner-city youngsters.
- Many disadvantaged children live in inadequate housing in segregated communities.
- Over half of all disadvantaged children are slum-dwelling black children.
- When inner-city children enter school, their communicative abilities are different from those of middle class children; according to Jones (1972), these varying speech and language patterns sometimes result in misunderstandings in oral communication.
- Motivation and educational achievement among these children are generally regarded as low.

Although Jones acknowledges that the foregoing characteristics have been profiled through numerous studies, she cautions that the speech-language pathologist should not generalize them to all inner-city children. The speech-language pathologist should look beyond these differences and attempt to understand the child in terms of his or her cultural background.

Second, the speech-language pathologist must learn to differentiate between speech and language pathologies and speech and language differences related to cultural factors. Children presenting the latter should not be regarded as "too lazy, stupid, careless, or stubborn to speak correctly" (Jones, 1972, p. 25).

Third, the speech-language pathologist should be aware of inexpensive or free services for those children requiring dental and medical services. Referral and follow-up work should be pursued vigorously when medical problems may be related to the child's communicative disorder. As speech-language pathologists in Baltimore discovered, when a need is demonstrated, the demand for medical services may result in the provision of appropriate services.

The fourth important component of successful intervention with inner-city children is the speech-language pathologist's ability to work with the parents of these children. The speech-language pathologist must realize that not all parents will be able to participate in the therapeutic process. Nevertheless, parent education should be included in the total program.

Fifth, the speech-language pathologist must have confidence that the children can profit from therapy and must then provide appropriate experiences to ensure some success. Sixth, accurate records must be kept on these children. Because of their high mobility rate, it is essential that all records be current so that when children transfer to other schools, there will be no interruption of services. Finally, Jones states that speech-language pathologists should not feel threatened when a child does not respond to therapy. Any number of factors, unrelated to the speech-language pathologist or the therapeutic approach, may affect the child's performance.

In summary, the speech-language pathologist, whether black or Caucasian, can be successful in working with inner-city children if he or she respects and demonstrates concern for these students. As Jones notes and as the foregoing discussion indicates, the role of the speech-language pathologist in dealing with culturally disadvantaged children presenting communicative differences is not entirely clear. Nevertheless, the school speech-language pathologist should be cognizant of appropriate assessment, intervention, and referral strategies in order to provide effective services to them.

Service Delivery to Indian Children

Historically, Indian children have been an underserved population. Recognizing that language experiences are prerequisite to successful entry into school and hypothesizing that some Indian children lacked these experiences, Canadian researchers (1969) undertook a four-week summer enrichment program. According to the researchers, good spoken language is not stressed by Indians, and they lack facility in reading. Further, Indian children display many characteristics of educationally disadvantaged children in that they lack self-confidence, do not come from educationally stimulating environments, are frequently undernourished, and display reduced language skills. A program was devised by the researchers to attack these deficiencies.

Following the four-week program, which emphasized language development, posttests revealed that the eight preschoolers involved had made significant improvement. The study indicated "that within the language areas assessed, a dramatic improvement in disadvantaged children's verbal patterns can be realized in a short period of time by actively involving the children in specific and well planned language experiences" (Mickelson & Galloway, 1969, p. 190). The authors further suggested that, without directed intervention, it is doubtful that the children's language would have improved.

Berman (1976) has reported on her experiences with Sioux Indian children in North Dakota. There she found families struggling with economic problems (the estimated mean annual income in 1972 was $3,000), social problems (including substandard housing, a high incidence of alcoholism, juvenile crime, and child neglect), medical problems, and educational problems. The educational difficulties were reflected by the fact that approximately 50 percent of all children who entered high school did not graduate. This was related, in part, to the utilization of traditional curricular programming; special education was not incorporated until 1971.

In August of 1972, Berman established her speech-language program. Supported by federal grant funding, she was able to order all the equipment she needed. Her speech room was located in a dormitory (many students lived in the dormitories during the week) near the elementary and high schools.

Screening and teacher referrals revealed that 79 of the 763 children and adolescents required speech-language services. During the next year, Berman's case load was reduced to 33 students. Only four of these students presented isolated articulatory disorders; the remainder had disorders of language in isolation or in combination with articulation. Three additional children had cleft palates, one was cerebral palsied, and six were mentally retarded. Berman also conducted language stimulation classes in the two kindergartens.

Discussing problems that she encountered, Berman mentioned that there was a space shortage. Additionally, the children involved in therapy did not practice outside of therapy sessions, and parental cooperation was poor. Berman rectified this situation in 1973 when she trained five aides to provide additional assistance to the children; four student aides were later trained to work with students with interdental lisps.

In reviewing the situation on the Standing Rock Sioux Reservation, Berman emphasized points made by Mickelson and Galloway. The Indian children were generally shy and quiet; they also exhibited reduced vocabularies. Although problems were encountered, the author indicated that the children did profit from intervention. She recommended that speech-language pathologists working with Indian children should have a good understanding of language disorders.

Although additional provision of services to Indian children may have occurred prior to 1975, the enactment of PL 94-142 had particular implications for these students. This previously underserved population is entitled to free appropriate educational services, including speech and language programming. Speech-language pathologists who work with Indian children have an obligation to familiarize themselves with the culture and environment of the reservation, as well as with the expectations of Indian children and their parents. The ways in which these children differ from the average—like the characteristics that distinguish any culturally different children—must be taken into account in assessment, intervention, and referral.

Discussion

It is acknowledged that culturally different children do not always reside in inner cities or on reservations, nor are they always black or Indian. They may come also from rural areas or from the suburbs. Regardless of people's origins or places of residence, their educational, social, and vocational success tends to be related to their ability to conform to a "standard" pattern of behavior. If a child is unable to employ "standard" language patterns, he may be impeded in attaining such success.

The responsibilities of the speech-language pathologist in working with children displaying culturally different communication patterns are still undefined. One important concern involves the goals that are appropriate for such children. The involvement of parents and of the child himself in establishing specific objectives and goals should help to clarify this concern. In addition, the methods of assessment utilized with culturally different children must be carefully selected. Intervention strategies should also be adapted to the needs and motivations of the students. A long-term contract plan may be ineffective with a child who does not know the origin of his or her next meal. Finally, the speech-language pathologist dealing with communicatively disordered children must be aware of referral opportunities. To suggest that parents of such a student take their child to an otolaryngologist might produce negative results; to refer them to a free clinic for equivalent services would probably be more useful.

SERVICE DELIVERY TO INCARCERATED YOUTHS

PL 94-142, the Education for All Handicapped Children Act of 1975, specifies that speech, language, and hearing services must be provided to handicapped students in institutions and hospitals as well as to those in private and public schools. For some speech-language pathologists, working with delinquent youths may not be unusual. For the others, the idea of providing services within the confines of an institution may be somewhat threatening.

Little research is available in the area of communicative disorders among juvenile delinquents. One early study was conducted by Cozad and Rousey (1966). These researchers hypothesized that the incidence of communicative disorders would be higher among delinquent youths than among those not so identified. Of the 300 subjects involved in audiometric testing, 24 percent were identified as hearing impaired. Speech disorders were diagnosed in 58.3 percent of the 252 youthful offenders evaluated. Since no attempt was made to assess linguistic abilities, it may be assumed that this incidence figure would have been greater had language been evaluated.

A few years later, the communicative abilities of 119 male juvenile delinquents incarcerated in the Missouri Training School for Boys (MTSB) were assessed (Taylor, 1969). Tests of language, hearing, and articulation were administered, and clinical judgments were made regarding voice and fluency. Only 19 of the youths evaluated demonstrated communicative abilities within the normal range. Among the 84 percent with communicative disorders, the predominant disability was in the area of language. This type of disorder was found in 50 of the boys, and an additional 41 demonstrated disordered language and concomitant problems. On the basis of these findings, it was recommended that an evaluative–habilitative program be established at the Training School.

Irwin (1977), a part-time speech-language pathologist at the MTSB, replicated the preceding study with some variation in the testing procedures. Irwin evaluated 100 boys in residence at the MTSB and found that 32 subjects had adequate communicative abilities. Linguistic disorders in isolation or in combination with other deviations were noted in 57 youths. The total incidence was 68 percent. Despite differences in incidence figures, Irwin concluded that a need did exist for the provision of services in that institution.

In a later article, Irwin has outlined the speech and language pathology program in place at the MTSB (1979). By 1979, the institution had put into operation a *positive peer culture program* (PPC). This technique relies on the residents to modify their behaviors, attitudes, and values as a result of their relationships with each other, rather than under the direction of an adult worker. Subgroups are formed within the institution, each consisting of nine boys. In group meetings, the youths and an adult leader analyze the behavior of each participant in terms of the reactions and behavioral patterns that are troublesome to other members. The boys learn to discuss their problems and share their concerns. When eventually a group member is to leave the institution, the group must agree to his release.

The need for a speech and language program at the MTSB was suggested by three factors. Initially, the relatively high incidence of youths presenting communicative disorders indicated that such a program was warranted. In addition, it was assumed that the resident with a communicative disorder might be ineffective in the PPC program, which relies heavily on group discussion and interaction. Finally, it is conceivable that a youth's adjustment after release from the institution could depend on his communicative abilities.

Residents are evaluated for the speech and language program by the speech-language pathologist; presumably all youths are seen shortly after admission to the institution. The Utah Test of Language Development and the Peabody Picture Vocabulary Test are the tools employed to evaluate language. Articulatory skills are assessed by means of the Goldman-Fristoe Test of Articulation. Hearing sensitivity is evaluated, and clinical judgments of fluency and voice are made. When necessary, boys are referred for additional testing or examination.

When a boy is included in the therapy program, members of the group are informed of his problem, of the intervention strategies to be used, and of the desired outcome. The group members then monitor the boy's progress, reinforce appropriate behavior, and provide feedback to the speech-language pathologist. Monitoring by group members is possible on a 24-hour per day basis. Charts are sometimes kept, and a weekly evaluation of the group member under observation is made by the group. Reinforcement is also provided by the group. According to Irwin, the intrinsic value derived from the recognition by other group members improves the self-concept of the youth involved in therapy. Feedback from a well-informed group may be very valuable. Irwin reported that some group members have made suggestions that proved helpful in the remedial process.

Staff members are also involved in therapy. A logbook is kept on each boy, and staff members can be informed of a boy's problem and progress through entries made by the speech-language pathologist. Conversely, by referring to the log, the speech-language pathologist remains abreast of the treatment strategies employed by other staff members. In this way, all members of the professional and treatment staff can be consistent in behavior management. Additionally, staff members are able to reinforce targeted speech and/or language behaviors and monitor a boy's progress.

As noted earlier, a boy must have the approval of his group (as well as the cottage committee) before he can be released from the institution. Although it is doubtful that a youth's dismissal would be postponed if he had not overcome his communicative disorder, consideration is given to the amount of progress that has taken place. According to Irwin, the youth must demonstrate responsibility for his behavior prior to being released.

In summary, Irwin acknowledges that some problems exist in providing services to incarcerated youths. Appropriate materials are somewhat difficult to locate. In addition, many questions remain to be answered. For example, What is the effect of therapeutic intervention? Do the youths perceive therapy to be of value, especially after their release? How does the treatment staff view the speech, language, and hearing program? According to Irwin, answers to these and other questions may be important in solving the problems of juvenile delinquency.

The author presented a model for speech-language services for both youthful and adult offenders in *Federal Probation* (Taylor, 1980). In recognition of the fact that the indeterminate nature of a youth's incarceration limits the possibilities of long-range intervention, this model emphasizes evaluation and postrelease follow-up.

The initial contact between the speech-language pathologist and the offender is during the intake process. The preliminary meeting is the equivalent of the screening procedure in the school setting. During informal conversation with the youth, any problems in the areas of articulation, voice, fluency, language, or hearing can be identified. If there are no observable disorders, a report to that effect can be entered in the intake summary. If, on the other hand, a communicative disorder is suspected, a complete evaluation should be conducted as soon as possible. Expeditious referrals are imperative, owing to the indeterminate nature of sentencing procedures.

Appropriate diagnostic tools for adolescents are difficult to locate. Irwin utilizes the Goldman-Fristoe Test of Articulation (GFTA). Although the utilization of a picture test with this age group may seem inappropriate, the unfortunate truth is that many incarcerated youths are unable to respond to a sentence test or even a word list. Since PL 94-142 requires that two modes of assessment be employed, some type of formal tool must be used. The ingenious speech-language pathologist in an institution might develop a test using photographs of objects and actions of greater interest to adolescents than those depicted by the GFTA. It goes without saying that the major concern in evaluating articulation is the adequacy of conversational speech; formal single-word testing or contextual testing serves only to confirm the presence and nature of the suspected disorder.

With reference to language, even fewer tools are available. In addition to the Utah Test of Language Development, the Peabody Picture Vocabulary Test, and the Screening Test of Adolescent Language, the speech-language pathologist may also secure and analyze a language sample. A problem in this area is the determination of the appropriateness of linguistic patterns. Should they be judged in relation to those of other boys confined in institutions or in relation to standard linguistic patterns? Institutional residents tend to develop their own jargon, and standard tests fail to decode these differences. Therefore, assessment in the area of language is difficult.

The evaluation of a boy with a fluency disorder can be facilitated by the institutional setting. Frequently, the speech-language pathologist must rely on client reports of stuttering behavior outside of the therapy situation. The confined youth's speech can be assessed not only in the traditional one-to-one situation but also as he interacts with peers in the classroom and during his work assignment. Interaction with staff members can also be observed. If group meetings are held, as in the PPC program, additional opportunities are provided. In general, a comprehensive description of the boy's fluency disorder can be achieved; as a result, the treatment plan may be equally comprehensive and appropriate.

As noted at the outset, boys with vocal or hearing disorders may require medical attention, and referrals should be expedient. It may be possible for some improvement to be made if medical clearance (in the case of boys with vocal disorders) is obtained quickly. The youth who has been seen by an audiologist and an otologist may respond to therapeutic intervention even during a brief confinement.

Once the comprehensive evaluation has been completed, the speech-language pathologist should be able to devise an appropriate IEP. Although parental involvement in the IEP preparation may be difficult, treatment staff members, the boy's teacher(s), and other institutional personnel should participate; the youth, himself, should also be involved. Implementation of the IEP should begin following the IEP conference.

In the event that the goals established in the IEP are not reached during the boy's confinement, all information collected by the speech-language pathologist is forwarded to the local education agency in the youth's home community. Thus, if the boy returns to his home school, his records are available to the school speech-language pathologist, and a duplication of effort can be avoided. By the same token, if the youth enters the institution with a current IEP, evaluation and preparation of such a plan should be unnecessary.

Intervention must not be terminated when a boy is dismissed from the correctional facility. Those juveniles who return to school should receive continued therapy in the educational setting. Alternative opportunities for therapy should be located for youths who do not pursue additional education. The institutional speech-language pathologist must be aware of appropriate facilities in the boy's community and should make every effort to ensure that adequate follow-up is provided. Again, the indeterminate nature of sentencing makes thorough follow-up extremely important.

Although many speech-language pathologists may feel ill-prepared to deal with incarcerated delinquents, at least two states specify compliance with PL 94-142 in their plans for special education. Both Kansas and Illinois allude to the provision of such services to youths confined to correctional institutions. In many cases, it will be the school speech-language pathologist who is assigned to the facilities. Assignments of this nature should be viewed as a challenge to the speech-language pathologist. They provide the professional with opportunities to deal with many aspects of a youth's behavior and to share in the experience of assisting that youth to become an independent and productive citizen.

Service Delivery in Secondary Schools

Another underserved population in the older age range includes adolescents in high school. Although larger districts are able to provide service to students at this level, it is doubtful whether smaller districts, which have difficulty servicing preschool and elementary students adequately, can assign speech-language pathologists to work in high schools. In any event, there is little convincing evidence to document the necessity of extensive intervention at the high school level. Finally, current educational programming at the high school level sometimes precludes the provision of appropriate speech and language services. Nevertheless, the mandate of PL 94-142 is that therapy be provided to all children and youths with communicative disorders. Therefore, consideration of programming at the secondary level is warranted.

Neal (1976), in an attempt to determine the status of speech and language programs in secondary schools, sent a questionnaire to 250 randomly selected public school speech-language pathologists. Identifying information and data on program management were requested. Essentially, the survey dealt with the similarities and differences between elementary and secondary school speech-language programs.

Of the 85 questionnaires returned, only 64 could be included in the final tabulation. Of the respondents, 23 worked in suburban school systems, 21 each in inner and rural areas, and 7 speech-language pathologists were in other settings. (Apparently, several respondents worked in more than one environment.) The majority of the speech-language pathologists held master's degrees (89 percent), and a similar majority had earned the Certificate of Clinical Competence from ASHA (81 percent).

When asked if they felt academically prepared to work with adolescents, 18 percent responded that they were well trained; 55 percent felt that their preparation was adequate; 18 percent felt inadequately trained; and 10 percent reported that they had received no training at all for the age level they were serving. The overwhelming majority recommended that additional course work and therapeutic experience, both in clinical and school settings, be provided at the preprofessional and professional training levels.

In investigating procedures followed at the secondary level, Neal found that teacher referral was the most popular method of case finding. Traditional itinerant scheduling was employed by 75 percent of the 53 speech-language pathologists working with secondary level students. A similar percentage (77.8 percent) indicated that intermittent scheduling was the most effective method, 14.8 percent favored intensive cycle scheduling, and 7.4 percent recommended other methods.

The 29 secondary level speech-language pathologists reported that the average number of students seen in individual sessions each week was just over 5, whereas 11.69 adolescents were seen for group therapy. Individual sessions averaged 28.77 minutes in length, and the average group session was over 30 minutes long. For the most part, both individual and group therapy sessions were held only once each week.

Although 23.8 percent of the responding speech-language pathologists felt that therapy techniques employed in primary and secondary schools were similar, 71.6 percent indicated that there were significant differences. Modification and development of techniques were reported by the majority of the speech-language pathologists. The professionals further reported that the techniques were more individualized at the secondary level; the emotional status of the student at this level influenced therapy to a greater extent.

In responding to questions about therapy materials, the speech-language pathologists indicated that clinician-prepared materials are more prevalent at the secondary level and that these materials frequently relate to information being covered in the students' classes. Interestingly enough, few speech-language pathologists employed electronic devices with high school students; further, they did not feel that more time was spent in therapy preparation even though adaptation of materials was required.

The final area covered by the questionnaire comprised factors affecting programmatic success. The speech-language pathologists rated students' motivation, attendance, and perception of other people's attitudes toward them and their problems as the factors most affecting the success of the program. Cooperation of classroom teachers, parents, and administrative personnel was among the least important factors. According to Neal, these findings may indicate that parents and teachers play smaller roles in the therapeutic process as the student gets older. On the other hand, the opinions of other persons assume increasing importance.

Fellows (1976) has discussed her perception of the role of the speech-language pathologist working in the high school setting. She considers the difficulties encountered in convincing students that they will benefit from therapy and in locating materials suitable for use with this age group. According to Fellows, case selection is crucial. Students must understand evaluative procedures and results and must be included in planning intervention strategies. They must also be convinced that therapy will be worthwhile; the value of therapy is sometimes difficult to explain to a student who has been exposed to the game-like approach utilized at the elementary school level. If, after these subjects have been discussed, the adolescent does not want to participate in therapy, his decision is accepted and respected. A negative decision does not, however, preclude his involvement in therapy at a later time.

Scheduling at the secondary level presents some problems. If students do not have study hall and must miss content courses, it is important to schedule them during classes absence from which will not appreciably affect academic performance. Fellows also indicates that utilization of class related materials will make therapy more attractive. Students realize that they are improving communicative and academic skills concurrently. Classroom teachers can be instrumental in suggesting appropriate materials for inclusion in therapy sessions.

The speech-language pathologist in the high school frequently provides services to special education students. Functional work with currency will improve mathematical skills. In order to improve spatial orientation and vocabulary, Fellows suggests that maps, globes, and driver education manuals be employed.

In general, materials including information considered important by the student should be utilized. As noted in Neal's discussion, procedures should be highly individualized.

REFERENCES

American Speech and Hearing Assocation. *Standards and guidelines for comprehensive language, speech, and hearing programs in the schools.* Washington, D.C., 1973–1974.

American Speech and Hearing Association Subcommittee on Housing of the Committee on Speech and Hearing Services in the Schools. ASHA recommendations for housing of speech services in the schools. *Asha,* 1969, *11,* 181–182.

Berman, S. S. Speech and language services on an Indian reservation. *Language, Speech, and Hearing Services in Schools,* 1976, *7,* 56–60.

Black, M. *Speech correction in the schools.* Englewood Cliffs: Prentice-Hall, 1964.

Bountress, N. G. Attitudes and training of public school clinicians providing services to speakers of black English. *Language, Speech, and Hearing Services in Schools,* 1980, *11,* 41–49.

Cozad, R., & Rousey, C. Hearing and speech disorders among delinquent children. *Corrective Psychiatry and Journal of Social Therapy,* 1966, *12,* 250–255.

Fellows, J. B. The speech pathologist in the high school setting. *Language, Speech, and Hearing Services in Schools,* 1976, *7,* 61–63.

Howerton, G. E. What can be done about substandard space for speech correction programs. *Language, Speech, and Hearing Services in Schools,* 1973, *4,* 95–96.

Irwin, D. L. A comparative study of the disorders of communication among incarcerated delinquents: Further implications for remedial speech and language programs. *The Journal of the Missouri Speech and Hearing Association,* 1977, *10,* 27–33.

Irwin, D. L. A speech and language pathology program for incarcerated delinquents. *The Journal of the Missouri Speech and Hearing Association,* 1979, *12,* 10–17.

Jones, S. A. The role of the public school speech clinician with the inner-city child. *Language, Speech, and Hearing Services in Schools,* 1972, *3,* 20–29.

Knight, H., Hahn, E. S., Ervin, J. C., & McIssac, G. The public school clinician: Professional definition and relationships. *Journal of Speech and Hearing Disorders Monograph Supplement 8,* 1961, 10–21.

Luper, H. L., & Ainsworth, S. Speech correction rooms in the public schools. *Exceptional Children,* 1955, *22,* 24, 38.

Mickelson, N. I., & Galloway, C. G. Cumulative language deficit among Indian children. *Exceptional Children,* 1969, *36,* 187–190.

Neal, W. R., Jr. Speech pathology services in the secondary schools. *Language, Speech, and Hearing Services in Schools,* 1976, *7,* 6–16.

North Dakota Department of Public Instruction. *Special Education in North Dakota Guidelines III: Programs for Students with Language, Speech, and Hearing Disorders in the Public Schools.* 1977.

Taylor, J. S. Speech-language services for youthful and adult offenders. *Federal Probation,* 1980, *44,* 37–41.

Taylor, J. S. *The communicative abilities of juvenile delinquents: a descriptive study.* Doctoral dissertation, University of Missouri—Columbia, 1969.

8

The School Speech-Language
Pathologist's Role
in Parent Counseling
and Supervision

It is now the rule rather than the exception that school clinicians take pride in their work, use highly efficient methods of organization and management of their programs, and possess clinical skills at least equal to those of their colleagues in other employment environments. (Van Hattum, 1976, p. 59)

Throughout the years, the attributes and responsibilities of competent public school speech-language pathologists have received consideration from a number of sources. Black (1964) has described the "speech therapist's" responsibilities in terms of direct services; professional relationships with administrators, classroom teachers, guidance personnel, and colleagues; and involvement with parents. The "speech clinician's" roles as professional person, educational team member, consultant, counselor, and researcher have also been explored (Van Hattum, 1969). With the advent of state and federal legislation, the responsibilities of the school speech-language pathologist have expanded. Counseling and supervisory activities now consume additional time. This chapter describes specific roles and responsibilities. Emphasis is given to those activities now increasing in importance.

THE ROLES OF THE SPEECH-LANGUAGE
PATHOLOGIST: AN OVERVIEW

Over 25 years ago, Powers (1956) presented a method for evaluating the work of the effective public school "speech therapist." The efficiency of the professional in the areas described in the following outline was to be rated as excellent, satisfactory, or unsatisfactory:

• Program organization, including case finding, case selection, scheduling, and maintenance of records
• Evaluative procedures, including knowledge of appropriate tools and of their diagnostic reliability
• Direct intervention, including skills in managing students, planning and executing therapy, and evaluating therapy results
• Relationships with colleagues within the school system, including building principals, classroom teachers, administrators, and other school personnel; and with parents and other professional persons and groups within the community
• Personal characteristics, including appearance, communicative ability, personality, intellectual functioning, and cultural attainment
• Professional ethics and attitudes, including attitudes toward clients, their families, and colleagues, and dedication to the profession

According to Powers, the effective speech specialist rates high in all of these areas, and utilization of this outline by speech-language pathologists, their supervisors, and school administrators should assist in assessing efficiency in specific roles. Further, Powers suggested, university professors might refer to this outline as they devise courses for students preparing to enter the schools, and students in training might consult it as they assess their interests in working in the school setting.

A need to distinguish the functions of the school speech-language pathologist from those of the instructional staff was identified in the early 1960s, leading to a statement by the Committee on Definitions of Public School Speech and Hearing Services of the American Speech and Hearing Association (1962). With regard to to the professional environments in which speech-language pathologists work, the statement indicates that although settings vary, the responsibilities of the professional remain the same. According to the Committee, "The nature of the services provided and the educational requirements necessary for clinical competence do not vary in any fundamental way for the different employment context" (American Speech and Hearing Association Committee on Definitions of Public School Speech and Hearing Services, 1962, p. 99).

The statement differentiates between the instructional role of the curriculum-oriented school personnel and the noninstructional role of the school speech-language pathologist. The former are trained to provide instruction based on a specific curriculum. Speech-language pathologists, on the other hand, provide diagnostic and remedial services based on the specific communicative disorder presented by the individual child. Curricular materials are not related to these activities.

The Committee further recommended that certification boards be helped to understand that preparation for school employment should not require extensive training in education. The statement suggested that the academic preparation of teachers and speech-language pathologists is specialized but not similar. Students in training should not be overburdened by the course work in education at the expense of training in their major area of interest.

The professional affiliations of speech-language pathologists were also addressed by the Committee. When speech-language pathologists are regarded as instructional personnel, they are often required to affiliate with general educational organizations rather than with speech and hearing associations. Instead, these professionals should be encouraged to read technical journals and to attend meetings devoted to the study of communicative disorders.

Finally, the Committee considered the issue of case load. In order to provide services that meet the needs of communicatively disordered children, it was recommended that case load size be reduced. Again, recognition that the role of the speech-language pathologist differs from that of instructional staff is necessary.

In an effort to define the functions of the public school speech-language pathologist even more concisely, the American Speech and Hearing Association Committee on Speech and Hearing Services in the Schools (1964) prepared an additional statement. Specifically, the Committee addressed the role of the speech-language pathologist in speech improvement. One concern was that speech-language pathologists not become so involved in speech improvement that they would be unable to provide services to children with handicapping disorders. The former group of children, those involved in speech improvement, are students whose communicative abilities are within normal limits but who can benefit from some assistance. The school speech-language pathologist should not service those children directly but rather should act as a consultant to the classroom teacher. It is students with handicapping conditions who require the direct services of the speech-language pathologist. Again, the Committee emphasized that the speech-language pathologist performs the same duties in the schools as he or she would in any other setting. These responsibilities include identification, evaluation, and execution of a program based on the child's communicative disorder. Speech improvement is not one of these responsibilities, but the speech-language pathologist may act in a consultative role in this area.

The School Speech-Language
Pathologist's Role in Education

Ainsworth (1964), in a follow-up article, discussed the public school "speech clinician" and queried whether a professional in that setting should be considered a "participant" or a "separatist." The "separatist" view perceives the speech-languag pathologist as a professional who functions cooperatively in a specific setting. Along with that viewpoint goes the spoken or unspoken fear that the effectiveness of the speech-language pathologist might be neutralized if he or she became too involved in the educational program. The "participant" point of view assumes that the speech-language pathologist should not only perform a service in the school setting but should also make a contribution to the educational program. "In addition to conducting himself appropriately as a speech pathologist, this specialist is obligated to carry out this work in such a way that it will reinforce and, in turn, be reinforced by appropriate educational activities in the total school program" (Ainsworth, 1964, pp. 495–496). Thus, the responsibilities of school speech-language pathologists in the schools are different from their responsibilities in other work environments.

In considering these points of view, Ainsworth discussed the speech-language pathologist's responsibilities to the child, the institution, and the profession. The primary responsibility of the professional is to the client. Speech-language pathologists who view themselves as "participants" can take advantage of many opportunities to reinforce the therapeutic process and, therefore, to meet the needs of the child. Working with teachers, the speech-language pathologist can suggest appropriate activities and demonstrate how they relate to the total educational program. On the other hand, the "separatist" who chooses to work outside of the educational program misses these opportunities and, as a result, deprives children of the total services they deserve.

Participation in the total educational program also evokes the cooperation of administrators and teachers. These persons learn to understand and respect the work of the school speech-language pathologist as the latter demonstrates appreciation of their roles. Speech-language pathologists who separate themselves from the total program may not inspire such support. The resulting lack of team effort will certainly not work in favor of the communicatively disordered child.

Finally, school speech-languguage pathologists must realize that they represent the school in the eyes of the parents regardless of whether they choose to or not. Parents realize that their tax dollars are responsible for the presence of the speech-language pathologist in the school and that he or she is there to provide a service.

Regarding the speech-language pathologist's responsibility to the institution, Ainsworth comments that anyone affiliated with a specific institution should be expected to contribute to its goals. In order for school speech-language pathologists to make such a contribution, they must understand both the social and educational objectives of a school. Some knowledge of the problems inherent in the school setting is also necessary. Further, the speech-language pathologist should perceive the way in which speech-language pathology services contribute to the total educational program. In order to function effectively within the school setting, the speech-language pathologist must be a "participant" rather than a "separatist."

Finally, speech-language pathologists have a responsibility to their profession, and their demeanor in the school setting will influence the attitudes of others toward the field of speech-language pathology. Those speech-language pathologists who choose to function as "separatists" in the schools do not contribute positively to the public's concept of the profession. It is necessary for the professional to participate cooperatively in all settings, including the schools. Such participation should not interfere with the speech-language pathologist's primary responsibility to the children but rather should allow him or her to contribute to the institution and the profession as well.

The School Speech-Language Pathologist's Status in the Profession

Another problem for school speech-language pathologists is that their training is often inappropriate and inadequate. The effective speech-language pathologist in the schools must be knowledgeable in both program management and therapeutic intervention. The majority of public school children present articulatory disorders, and the speech-language pathologist is expected to work with these students in groups, with inadequate materials and in restricted space. By contrast, the student in training may see one to five clients per week, and these individuals sometimes present complex communicative disorders. The work area is functionally appropriate, and current materials and equipment are available. Clearly, the two situations are dissimilar, and the college experience does not fully prepare students to work in the school setting.

Another problem arises from the perception of the field the training program gives the student in training and the perception of the school system has of the speech-language pathologist. Clinical methods and experiences are provided to the student while in training; on the job, however, the speech-language pathologist is expected to be assimilated into an educational environment. School speech-language pathologists have reason to feel that their training is inappropriate.

Inadequacy in training is also identified in lack of preparation for program management. Van Hattum suggests that this area of training is sometimes covered in a two-hour course taught by someone who is inexperienced or whose experience was obtained many years ago. Moreover, he indicates that the teaching of academic theory, although critical, must not preclude training in practical application and program management. According to Van Hattum, it is remarkable that school speech-language pathologists are as competent as they are, considering their lack of preparation.

An important problem addressed by Van Hattum relates to the status afforded public school speech-language pathologists. Professionals in the schools tend to believe that neither their professional colleagues nor university training programs have respect for them. This latter view was reinforced by the statement of an individual from a training program who said, "I question that they [public school speech-language pathologists] are engaged in a clinical practice oriented to an individual and his unique disability. Those I have known are not suited by training, education, or inclination to be that kind of a clinician" (Van Hattum 1966, p. 238). Statements such as this certainly give the school speech-language pathologist cause to be defensive. As Van Hattum suggests, this kind of criticism is professionally unethical.

Although Van Hattum discussed roles already described by others, he did address an issue that still confronts the profession today. Is the school speech-language pathologist one rung down on the professional ladder from those working in hospitals, community centers, or university clinics? In order to determine how school speech-language pathologists would answer that and other questions, Weaver (1968) conducted a survey of 318 professional employed in the schools. A total of 192 responses to the mailed questionnaire were returned. The respondents' mean age was 34 years, and their years of school experience ranged from 1 to 41 years, with the mean a little over 8 years. Only 14 percent of the respondents were male.

One of the tasks requested in the questionnaire was a ranking of the following professionals in order of importance: classroom teacher, public school speech-language pathologist, special education teacher, speech-language pathologist employed in a setting other than the schools, and college instructor. Of the respondents, 89 percent completed the ranking and rated the classroom teacher well ahead of the other professionals. The school speech-language pathologist was ranked second, followed by college instructor, speech-language pathologist working outside of the schools, and special education teacher. If these results may be generalized, it would appear that public school speech-language pathologists do not regard themselves as second class citizens when compared with colleagues engaged in other settings.

The respondents were also asked to assign a level of importance to the work of the school speech-language pathologist. Of the respondents, 41 percent considered that work to be of "highest importance"; 52 percent assigned a ranking of "significant importance." Only 1.5 percent considered therapy in the school setting to be of "average importance," and less than 1 percent assigned a ranking of "less than average importance" or "not very important." Of the respondents, 98.5 percent ranked these levels of importance.

When asked whether public school therapy was of primary or secondary importance, 76 percent chose "primary," 18 percent selected "secondary," and 6 percent did not respond. Additionally, 93 percent answered that they would choose public school work if they had it to do over again, 5 percent stated that they would not, and 2 percent were uncertain.

Weaver also sought to determine if school speech-language pathologists felt that national, state, and local professional organizations were representing them well. Of the respondents with masters' degrees, only 38 percent felt that ASHA represented their needs; 28 percent of the bachelor's level respondents agreed. The remainder of the respondents felt that they were not well represented. With regard to the representation of interests, 23 percent felt that ASHA was the organization that best represented public school speech-language pathologists, whereas 44 percent indicated that their particular state organizations were more effective. The remaining respondents either chose not to respond or identified other organizations.

The results of Weaver's investigation suggest that public school speech-language pathologists have a positive image of themselves and a good attitude toward their positions in the schools. This seems to contradict Van Hatttum's belief that public school persons regard themselves as second class professionals. The respondents were less positive when questioned about the effectiveness of the national organization (ASHA) in representing them and their interests.

In recognition of the needs of public school speech-language pathologists, in 1969 ASHA created the position of Associate Secretary for School-Clinic Affairs (Albritton, 1970). A mailing list of 12,500 speech-language pathologists who worked in the schools or had an interest in school programs was developed. In addition, in April 1970, the first edition of *Speech and Hearing Services in Schools* (later, *Language, Speech, and Hearing Services in Schools*) was distributed to all persons on the mailing list. This journal has been instrumental in helping school speech-langauge pathologists maintain professional currency and in keeping them informed about pertinent developments specifically related to the public school setting. The journal's establishment was a positive acknowledgement by ASHA of the unique needs of public school speech-language pathologists.

Bown (1971), when considering the expanding responsibilities of the school speech-language pathologist, questioned whether ASHA should be involved in defining the role that the professional should play or whether this task could be carried out more effectively by the school speech-language pathologists themselves, and/or their administrators or superiors. Although no conclusions were drawn, the author did reflect on the new roles that speech-language pathologist's might play. One such role would be as a resource teacher based in a single building. As another possibility, school speech-language pathologists might begin to concentrate their efforts on children with complex communicative disorders, while the paraprofessionals worked with children with mild articulatory defects. Increased attention to the total needs of language disordered children was also predicted by Bown. Finally, the school speech-language pathologist must recognize the need to function cooperatively with other professionals and to define his or her role as a team member.

Van Hattum (1976), after alluding to his previous article regarding the "defensive" speech-language pathologist in the schools, has discussed progress that has been made in the interim, and has projected role modifications for the future. Acknowledging the establishment of the Associate Secretary for School Affairs by ASHA and the publication of *Language, Speech and Hearing Services in Schools,* Van Hattum also notes that school speech-language pathologists have higher regard for themselves than previously. In order that this progress be maintained and additional strides be made, Van Hattum suggests that school speech-language pathologists might need to adjust their professional roles.

Greater efficiency in service delivery might result from the utilization of altered delivery systems. Both communication aides and tape recorded articulation programs could reduce the number of children being serviced directly by the speech-language pathologist, allowing that professional to provide more intensive therapy to students with complicated communicative disorders. Van Hattum also discusses increased participation in service delivery to children who have linguistic disorders and learning disabilities and who are mentally retarded. The author emphasizes that the speech-language pathologist's responsibility to the retarded child is the same as it is to the student with normal intelligence; the role played by the speech-language pathologist may be consultative or direct. In addition, the area of prevention is one to be entered more vigorously. Early childhood screenings and intervention, when necessary, may prevent the development of handicapping conditions. Finally, Van Hattum suggested that school speech-language pathologists might want to reexamine their lack of training in the teaching of reading and writing. By acquiring such skills, speech-language pathologists might incorporate these areas into their therapy, thus increasing their potential value to the total educational program.

Alluding to Ainsworth's separatist–participant dichotomy, Van Hattum concurs that the separatist position was inconsistent with appropriate therapeutic management in the school setting. The future, he says, may depend on a reevaluation of the role played by the school speech-language pathologist. Professionals in the schools must be prepared to modify their delivery systems and to expand into the area of the total communicative and educational processes.

Falck (1978) has emphasized the importance of the speech-language pathologist's role in integrating speech and language services into the educational program and in consulting with parents and teachers. Calling attention to the "participant" role, Falck discusses way in which the speech-language pathologist can work with teachers and parents to meet the needs of communicatively disordered children. The speech-language pathologist's expertise in facilitating interaction in IEP meetings and teacher and parent conferences was also stressed.

Recently, a new opportunity for involvement of the speech-language pathologist with nonhandicapped children was discussed by Dublinske (1979). Pursuant to PL 95-156, the Education Amendments of 1978, speech-language pathologists may participate in basic skill improvement programming for students whose oral communicative skills are not impaired but could be improved. Such involvement will permit increased interaction of the speech-language pathologist with teachers, greater input into the curriculum, and expansion of career possibilities.

In summary, the roles of the speech-language pathologist in the schools are changing. No longer are assessment and direct intervention the only responsibilities the speech-language pathologist has. Of increasing importance are the school speech-language pathologist's skills in parent counseling and supervision.

PARENT COUNSELING

Speech-language pathologists and parents have opportunities to interact in ways that are potentially beneficial to the child. Initially, the speech-language pathologist may interview the parent. Additional opportunities for interaction occur during the IEP meeting and in conferences designed to obtain information from the parents or to suggest methods of managing the child at home. In most instances, the conferences take place in the school building, although some speech-language pathologists prefer to visit parents at home. Group meetings may supplement individual conferences. After a general discussion of the problems of counseling parents of handicapped children, this section gives specific consideration to the counseling of parents of communicatively disordered students.

Counseling Parents of Exceptional Children

Stewart (1978) suggests that counseling parents of an exceptional child involves a helping relationship between those parents and a knowledgeable professional. This relationship should allow the professional to understand the parents' feelings, concerns, and problems. Further, "It is a learning process focusing upon the stimulation and encouragement of personal growth by which parents are assisted in acquiring, developing, and utilizing the skills and attitudes necessary for a satisfactory resolution to their problem or concern" (p. 22).* Finally, the counseling process should allow the parents to function fully as individuals, to be assets to their child, and to create a well-adjusted family unit. This appears to be a reasonable description of what counseling parents of exceptional children should be, and it is accepted as a working definition for this discussion.

Successful "helping" individuals appear to have certain attitudes and characteristics. According to Stewart (1978), the counselor must be interested in people and must accept them as worthy persons. Empathy is an important quality. "As one counsels with parents, we must have (or develop) an ability to, so far as humanly possible, understand their meanings and feelings" (p. 29). The counselor must possess sufficient security to be genuine and honest in the helping relationship and must be an attentive listener. Above all, counselors must be professional and ethical in their behavior. Not only must professionals handle confidential information discreetly; they must also recognize their limitations in the counseling role. Although these attitudes and characteristics are specified as necessary qualities for a counselor, they are also attributes of an effective speech-language pathologist.

The counseling process, itself, involves several phases. Stewart suggests that although the steps may fuse, six phases may be identified. The initial interview, or Phase 1, affords the counselor and counselee the first opportunity to relate to each other. During this interview, the problem may be stated and explored and plans can be made for the future. Next, in Phase 2, the nature of the counseling process is defined. In Phase 3, the counselor seeks to understand the client's needs and to express this understanding to the client. Solutions to the problem are explored in Phase 4 and a plan of action is devised in Phase 5. Finally, the sessions are terminated by mutual agreement. Stewart indicates that not all counseling relationships will follow this sequence nor include all steps but that it does represent the problem solving process.

Several techniques are employed by trained counselors in conducting sessions. Traditionally, these have included the directive, nondirective, and eclectic approaches. Using the directive approach, the counselor is an active participant in guiding the counselee. It is assumed that the counselor, by virtue of his or her training and experience, is qualified to advise the client, whose background in certain areas may be deficient. The parents of a handicapped child, for example, may not understand the problems presented by that child as well as the professional. Therefore, a directive approach is

---

*From *Counseling Parents of Exceptional Children* by J. C. Stewart. Columbus: Charles E. Merrill Publishing Company, 1978. Reprinted by permission.

employed by the counselor to obtain information and provide advice for child-management.

There are those who feel that the directive technique places undue emphasis on the counselor's role in problem solving. In fact, it is sometimes referred to as the counselor-centered approach. Further, directive counseling may encourage the client to become dependent on the counselor. In using this counseling strategy, one should exercise care in giving personal advice to the client. According to Stewart (1978), "A rule of thumb that can be followed is not to give advice unless it is in the form of tentative suggestions based upon solid expertise or in the form of possible alternatives that have been successfully tried out by other parents of exceptional children" (p. 52).

Although the nondirective or client-centered technique is most efficiently employed by professional counselors, some of these strategies may be utilized in counseling the parents of handicapped children. Basically, in this approach, the counselor views the client as possessing the ability to solve his or her own problems without the advice of the counselor. The professional's objective is to create a situation in which the client can identify and explore the problem objectively. In addition, the counselor must attempt to see the problem as the client views it and communicate this understanding to him or her. In order to achieve these goals, the counselor must listen attentively and reflect and clarify the client's attitudes and feelings.

As opposed to the directive technique, nondirective counseling tends to discourage client dependency since clients make their own decisions. Unfortunately, the fact that it is time consuming precludes extensive utilization of this strategy in the school setting.

The eclectic approach includes utilization of appropriate techniques from a variety of counseling strategies. The eclectic counselor believes that "a single orientation is limiting and that procedures, techniques, and concepts from many sources should be utilized to best serve the needs of the person seeking help" (Stewart, 1978, p. 55). Although this approach appears to be the most reasonable, there is some question as to whether a single counselor can become expert in all counseling strategies and capable of applying them effectively.

In summary, the traditional counseling techniques differ in terms of counselor involvement and in terms of the presenting problems to which they may be applied. Directive counseling revolves around the counselor and is appropriately applied in the educational, behavioral management, and vocational areas. In the nondirective approach, the role of the counselor is less prominent, and emphasis is placed on the problem solving abilities of the client. This technique is employed when the presenting problems are in the personal or social areas. Finally, eclectic counselors select strategies from directive, nondirective, and other approaches according to the needs of their clients. According to Stewart, the effective application of the method, rather than the method itself, is the critical factor.

One additional counseling technique is the behavioral or action strategy. This method recognizes that observation of behavior is the only certain way to determine whether change has occurred. Behavioral counseling "is a process involving a learning situation in which the counselee learns more appropriate behaviors" (Stewart, 1978, p. 59). Of concern to the counselor are the maladaptive behaviors, the supportive environmental contingencies, and the reinforcing stimuli that might be applied to alter the maladaptive behavior. These factors are explored in three phases. First, the client–counselor relationship is established. During the second phase, the counselor and client determine the approach to be taken and decide which techniques would be effective. In the third and final stage, the action planned in the second is taken and analyzed.

Behavioral counseling, because it has observable and measureable effects, is advantageous to both client and counselor. Conversely, one disadvantage is that the effective utilization of behavioral counseling depends upon the counselor's understanding of behavior theory; according to Stewart, many counselor are not sufficiently conversant with this theory and its application to employ it efficiently.

Stewart has also addressed specific issues related to the counseling process, including group counseling. When properly executed, group counseling allows the members to interact with others who have similar concerns and counseling goals. Counselors function in a group setting in much the same way they function in individual sessions. It is important that they create a situation in which group members feel secure and free to express themselves. Of equal importance is that all participants listen carefully and with understanding. The group might contain five to ten members, because, according to Stewart, it should be small enough to allow for personal interaction and large enough for group interaction. Group counseling with parents of exceptional children can be both efficient and effective when conducted by a properly trained professional.

The physical setting for counseling should be one that is conducive to communication. It should be comfortable and distraction-free. Privacy, both auditory and visual, is imperative. The arrangement of furniture is an important consideration. The directive counselor may wish to sit behind a desk, but the nondirective helper will probably avoid that type of physical barrier. It is suggested that the counselor experiment with various furniture arrangements until one that communicates the type of relationship he or she wishes to establish with the counselee is achieved.

Stewart also comments on the function of silence and nonverbal communication in the counseling process. Silence is sometimes feared by the inexperienced counselor, who feels that every moment should be filled with oral communication. "The counselor should realize that a great deal of communication takes place without sound and no rule exists that says all silence should be replaced with sound" (Stewart, 1978, p. 72). There are many reasons for silence, and the counselor should analyze and respect silent periods.

Similarly, the counselor should be alert to the nonverbal messages communicated by the counselee. One study involving a two-person conversation, for example, revealed that 65 percent of the social meaning was communicated nonverbally. Counselors should not only learn from the nonverbal communications of the client; they should also be aware of the nonverbal messages they themselves are relaying to the client. Such communications should not contradict the meaning they intend to convey, and in fact do convey in speech.

Finally, Stewart discusses the referral process. Professionals who counsel parents but who are not trained counselors must not attempt to handle situations beyond their level of competence. "Learning when and how to make referrals and determining what purpose will be served is almost as important as learning to counsel" (Stewart, 1978, p. 75). It is imperative that clients be included in the decision to refer and that they be responsible for making appointments for the new service.

Counseling Parents
of Communicatively Disordered Children

Speech-language pathologists, guided by several members of their profession, have recognized the need to improve their counseling skills. Webster has been particularly active in this area. In a 1966 article, she discusses counseling with parents of communicatively disordered children and defines the role of the speech-language pathologist as a counselor (Webster, 1966). Initially, assumptions regarding the parents are made. For example, it is assumed that because of the child's communicative disorder, the parents and their child are not communicating effectively with each other. It is further assumed that this lack of communication interferes with interpersonal relationships and that this, in turn, further complicates communication.

The relationship between the child's problem and the parents' behavior must be explored. Although it cannot be assumed that the parents caused the problem, anxiety on the part of both the child and parents may be evident as they communicate. Guilt is sometimes a factor; parents may wonder if they have contributed to their child's problem. It is with emotions such as these—and frequently with a lack of information about communicative disorders—that parents may enter the counseling situation.

The speech-language pathologist must realize that the parents are probably dealing with the problem as well as they can under the circumstances. Although speech-language pathologists can provide guidelines for managing a child, it is imperative that they not attempt to direct the child-rearing process. That is the parent's responsibility and privilege.

Lastly, it is assumed that the parents have the potential for growth and are motivated by the wish to do what is best for the child; to understand other people, including the child; to learn to communicate with their child on a more positive level; and to find fulfillment for themselves and their child. Concerning the last motivation, Webster emphasizes that parents must have an identity of their own. To deal with them strictly as parents, rather than as worthy human beings, would impede the counseling effort.

Webster cites three ways in which parents can benefit from counseling. First, counseling provides an opportunity for parents to discuss their feelings. Open discussion of fears and other emotions, motivations, and goals, is encouraged in the counseling situation, and such discussion should lead to more open communication between parents and their children. Second, the parents are given information regarding their childrens' communicative disorders. Not only are they provided with facts; the speech-language pathologist must also assist the parents in applying the information to their unique situations. Third and last, the speech-language pathologist should afford the parents opportunities to experiment with effective ways of improving communication. Webster (1966) cautions, however, that "the professional person's role is that of introduction and experimentation with tools; he cannot make others accept his ideas" (p. 334).* The "tools" Webster alludes to include a number of behavioral prescriptions for parents. For example, (1) The parents should try to understand what the child is feeling and to communicate this understanding to him or her; (2) the parents should learn to accept what the child is feeling even when the child's behavior is inappropriate; (3) the parents should provide opportunities for communication with the child when the latter will have their undivided attention, and these occasions should provide satisfaction and success for the child; and (4) the parents should attempt to communicate with the child at the child's level.

The role and attitudes of the counselor require consideration. According to Webster, the most important attitude is respect for the client. The counselor should also create a situation in which the client feels free to communicate; then the counselor should listen actively. The professional should also assist the parents in clarifying their feelings and ideas. An effective counselor must be knowledgeable about communicative disorders. Information provided to the parents must be accurate and must be presented in a relevant manner. The counselor must also be discreet in answering parents' questions. Some questions require direct answers; others, such as "What should I do if my child's friends tease him about his stuttering?", may often be referred back to the parent for consideration and resolution. Patience is another quality of a good counselor. Counselors should realize that any

---

*From "Parent Counseling by Speech Pathologists and Audiologists" by E. Webster. *Journal of Speech and Hearing Disorders,* 1966, *31,* 331–340. Reprinted by permission.

modification of attitude or behavior occurs slowly. Finally, Webster warns that the counselor must keep counseling sessions parent-centered rather than problem-centered. Positive aspects of daily living should be discussed as well as specific problems. The counselor should "be able to laugh with them [the parents] even as he is able to view their suffering with compassion" (Webster, 1966, p. 337).

Group counseling, according to Webster, is similar to individual conferences. Both require respect for the clients and open, attentive communication. In a group, however, the counselor must interact with more than one person at a time. An effective counselor will create a situation in which group members are supportive of each other; in effect, each may become a counselor. Group interaction may result in conflict between parents, however, and the counselor must be both alert to this possibility and prepared to resolve it. The effective group setting is one in which parents are permitted to disagree with each other but in which these conflicts do not interfere with the goal of counseling.

Since group interaction is necessary before the parents can learn from each other, the speech-language pathologist must encourage an atmosphere that permits open discussion. This will not occur if the professional chooses to lecture to the parents or if the speech-language pathologist is the dominant group member. As questions are asked, some should be answered directly and others should be opened for group discussion. The counselor should be aware that some members will not participate as readily as others. Their wishes to remain silent should be respected, although they may be encouraged to interact with the group. As Webster (1966) says, "It may be helpful to the clinician to remember that problem-solving can also begin in silence" (p. 339).

Concluding her article, Webster (1966) addresses a question sometimes asked by speech-language pathologists: "Can't the speech pathologist or audiologist do damage to parents by attempting to counsel with them?" (p. 339). If counseling is improperly done, the answer to that question is yes. The speech-language pathologist who is too authoritative, who provides inaccurate information, or who focuses on the child's problem while excluding parent's feelings may harm the parent. Conversely, the warm, accepting professional who listens and responds to the parent while providing him or her with sound information will be an effective counselor.

In a follow-up article, Webster (1968) elaborated on group counseling with particular regard for group discussion and role playing. Discussion constitutes the major portion of the group counseling process. Discussions should take place in a room containing comfortable furniture, arranged to allow all participants to see each other. The parents are encouraged to generate topics for discussion, but the speech-language pathologist serves as the discussion leader. During the discussions, the parents are helped to recognize the common problems they are experiencing and are encouraged to solve these problems together. At the same time, the speech-language pathologist is responsible for sharing information about communicative disorders with the less knowledgeable parents. The professional should also explain and demonstrate the tools (enumerated in Webster's earlier article) for improving child–parent communication.

Another technique to be utilized in group meetings with parents is role playing. The goals of role playing are to assist parents in understanding behavior and to permit them to experiment with different approaches to various situations. According to Webster, role playing consists of three phases. During the warm-up period, the speech-language pathologist helps group members define the situation, assigns roles, and assists the members in creating their roles. In the second phase, the situation is acted out and, finally, group members discuss what has happened.

Although role playing incorporates discussion in its first and third phases, it also requires actual bodily movement. This permits a demonstration of emotional behavior that may then be discussed. Because of this emotional component, role playing must be used cautiously. Further, this procedure lends itself to manipulation of the parents by the speech-language pathologist, something to be avoided. Webster suggests that speech-language pathologists should have participated in role playing previously so that they will have an understanding of the process and of its benefits and dangers. In the professional situation, however, they should direct, not participate in the role playing experience.

Emerick (1969) has addressed the issue of the parent interview, concentrating on information exchange rather than the counseling aspect of interaction between speech-language pathologist and parents. According to Emerick (1969), an interview "is a purposeful exchange of meanings between two persons, a directed conversation that proceeds in an orderly fashion to obtain data, to convey certain information and to provide release and support" (p.3).* The two participants in the interview should bring information to the meeting that will assist in understanding and helping the child.

Emerick identifies several problems in the interviewing process. One of these difficulties resides in the fears of the speech-language pathologist. Young professionals sometimes worry that parents will not recognize them as professionals because of their youth. This is usually an unfounded fear. Speech-language pathologists are also fearful that the parents will become defensive during the interview or ask unanswerable questions. Again, these situations do not occur frequently. When the speech-language pathologist experiences fear regarding an interview, the interview may be perceived as a threat or a challenge; obviously the latter reaction is preferable.

---

*From *The Parent Interview* by L. Emerick. Danville: The Interstate Publishers & Printers, Inc., 1969. Copyright 1969 by The Interstate Publishers & Printers, Inc. Used by permission.

When the speech-language pathologist perceives the parents as enemies, additional interviewing difficulties arise. Parents must be recognized as unique human beings rather than obstacles to therapeutic success. As Emerick points out, too often parents are blamed for the speech-language pathologist's lack of success with a child. "It is very easy to explain away our failures by criticizing the parents of our cases, especially when we sit in the relative safety of the broom closet [therapy room] each week on coordination day" (Emerick, 1969, p. 10). Acceptance of parents as participants in the therapeutic process will alleviate this problem.

Finally, Emerick identifies specific factors that interfere with communication during the interview. For example, (1) The parents may not remember critical information about the child; (2) emotional barriers may interfere with open communication; (3) the parents may conceal information; (4) the speech-language pathologist may deal ineffectively with parents from social classes different from his or her own; (5) language differences may cause a breakdown in communication; (6) the parents may be suspicious of the speech-language pathologist because he or she is associated with the school; and/or (7) the purpose of the interview may be unfocused. Speech-language pathologists should be aware of these potential interferences and avoid them whenever possible.

According to Emerick, there are three objectives of a diagnostic interview. The first is to obtain information. In preparing the parent for this task, the speech-language pathologist must define his or her role, as well as the role of the parents. The site of the interview is important for setting the tone of the session. It is Emerick's contention that the school setting is preferable to a home visit. Although many speech-language pathologists choose to open the interview with an assurance of confidentiality, Emerick suggests that the professional's manner alone should communicate such ethical behavior.

In seeking information, Emerick suggests that an interview guide be followed. Some speech-language pathologists utilize a questionnaire format, whereby the professional reads a question and the parent responds verbally. Emerick views such questionnaires as a barrier to effective interviewing or as a crutch for the inexperienced interviewer. The interviewing style (directive, nondirective, etc.) should be appropriate to the nature of the information sought. To obtain factual material, a directive approach may be required, whereas when emotionally charged information is discussed, a nondirective approach may be preferable.

Emerick feels that inexperienced interviewers are likely to make many strategic errors, and he singles out eleven of these as the most glaring. Table 8-1 describes these errors briefly.

The second objective of a diagnostic interview is to provide information to the parent. As Emerick points out, if professionals do not furnish accurate, nonemotional information regarding the child's communicative dis-

Table 8-1

Common Errors in Diagnostic Interviewing

The speech-language pathologist may

- Ask questions that can be answered yes or no

  This type of questioning tends to preclude discussions: an open-ended style is preferable.

- Bias an answer by the phrasing of a question

  The common example of this sort of questioning is the old line, When did you stop beating your wife?

- Talk too much

  Inexperienced interviewers are sometimes threatened by silence. By filling up pauses with conversation, they may miss opportunities to obtain valuable information.

- Dwell on etiology and physical symptoms, failing to respond to the parent's feelings and attitudes

  Some speech-language pathologists are so concerned with the pathology that they tend to ignore the emotional implications of the problem.

- Provide specific information too early in the interview

  Even though a parent may be laboring under a misconception, it is sometimes best to delay correcting such errors.

- Ask questions indirectly

  Sensitive questions should be asked directly. If, for example, the speech-language pathologist must know about the child's relationship with his or her siblings, the question should be phrased that way.

- Respond negatively to the parent's statements

  The interviewer must not impose his or her values on the parent's behavior or attitudes.

- Be incapable of delicately leading the interviewee who has wandered from the topic back to the discussion

  The interviewer should not attempt to do this by seeking new information but rather by returning to the answer the interviewee was giving when he or she began discussion tangential material.

- Accept superficial answers to questions

  There are numerous probes the interview can use to get beneath surface responses, and the speech-language pathologist should be familiar with these techniques.

- Attempt to obtain all information in one interview

  In some cases, the interviewee may reveal too much during the initial interview and then feel hostile or embarassed for having done so.

- Fail to take notes

  A record of the interview is imperative. Note, however, that the interviewee should always be told that notes are being taken or that the interview is being taperecorded. Such record taking rarely interferes with the interview.

SOURCE: Emerick, 1969.

order, the parents will probably seek answers from persons unqualified to provide such information. Although the language used by the speech-language pathologist must be nontechnical, it is important not to talk down to the parents. In imparting information to parents, Emerick suggests, the speech-language pathologist should (1) refrain from lecturing to parents; (2) use appropriate language and rephrase important points; (3) provide parents with something concrete to do; and (4) be direct, but pleasant, when discussing sensitive information.

The third and final objective of an interview is to provide release and support for the parents. One hopes that opportunities for the parents to ventilate will occur rather naturally throughout the interview. The speech-language pathologist should empathize with the parents when the latter discuss their feelings and problems. When emotional scenes occur—and they will—the speech-language pathologist has several options. He or she may leave the room, allowing the parents to regain their composure in privacy, or may attempt to change the subject. Both of these approaches, according to Emerick, may be construed as rejection by the interviewee. Perhaps the most humane way to deal with this type of situation is for the speech-language pathologist to communicate to the parents his or her understanding and acceptance of the parents' feelings. It should be understood that not all parents require an extensive interview. Frequently information sharing is the sole purpose of the meeting. In other instances, however, parents may need support and opportunities to vent their feelings.

Finally, Emerick suggests ways in which speech-language pathologists may improve their interviewing skills. First, the professional or student in training should do research in the area of interviewing and should explore the problems confronting parents of both normal and handicapped children. It is also suggested that role-playing experience in interviewing can be beneficial. Finally, Emerick recommends that the speech-language pathologist tape-record some actual interviews with parents and analyze these conferences with a supervisor or colleague.

Flynn (1978) has also discussed interviewing techniques and has identified several relevant facets of the interviewing procedures. With regard to the interview environment, Flynn notes that in addition to the privacy required for such a meeting, it is important that the area be clutter free. The client will have more confidence in the professional whose office is neat and whose records are carefully filed away. Chairs in the room should be placed at 90 degree angles so that eye contact is possible; this arrangement also allows for looking straight ahead when the client is attempting to think.

At the outset of the interview, Flynn suggests that the identity of the interviewee by verified so as to be certain that the correct person is present. She goes on to say that it is important that the speech-language pathologist avoid excessive casual conversation. According to Flynn, this might indicate to the counselee that the problem is either too serious or not serious enough to discuss. The time frame for the interview should also be established at the beginning of the session.

In discussing interviewing behaviors, Flynn comments on the function of silence. Like the other authors cited here, Flynn acknowledges that silence is a useful interviewing technique. She cautions, however, that too much silence may be discomforting to the client and may make the interviewer appear to be a cold person. Finally, Flynn notes the significance of closing the interview with a summary of the session. This allows for the correction of any misconceptions and identification of gaps in information obtained during the interview.

In a recent article, Webster and Cole (1979) discussed the speech-language pathologist's role as a leader of parent discussion groups. Essentially, the speech-language pathologist's function in this situation is to promote discussion by encouraging group members to talk; at the same time, the effective group leader is one who can remove himself from the leadership role. Regarding skills that the leader should have, the authors suggest that the professional should become adept at perceiving and identifying similarities among the group members. As the counselees recognize these similarities, group interaction is facilitated.

Topic selection has been addressed by Webster and Cole, who suggest that several options are available. The speech-language pathologist may select the topic, announce it, and have the parents discuss it. Another option is for the speech-language pathologist to suggest a topic, subject to parental approval. If the majority of the parents agree, the topic is discussed. As discussion takes place, additional topics will be suggested by parents. There are occasions, however, when the speech-language pathologist will identify a need to share specific information with the parents. When this occurs, it is the speech-language pathologist's ethical responsibility to schedule this as a discussion topic.

With regard to the provision of equal opportunities for parents to participate in group discussion, Webster and Cole again caution that not all group members will participate orally; some participation will be in silence. When grossly unequal participation occurs, the speech-language pathologist may want to taperecord meetings and analyze the participation of various members. This may assist in anticipating and correcting any inequities that may exist. Turn-taking may also be required when parents are competing for the opportunity to talk.

Evaluating the Effectiveness of Parent Counseling

Eisenstadt (1972) has looked at parental counseling from the parents' point of view. Parents whose children had been involved in extensive therapeutic programs were interviewed in order to ascertain their level of satisfaction with regard to parent–client–clinician relationships. Although most comments were favorable, several problem areas were identified. Some of these difficulties were the result of faulty communication between the parents and the speech-language pathologist; these problems might have been avoided if parental counseling had been more efficient.

Eisenstadt found, for example, that parents were unable to prepare their children for the initial diagnostic session because they, the parents, had no concept of what procedures would be followed. Prediagnostic preparation is particularly important when the evaluation will take place in a hospital setting. The consensus was that some indication of the nature of the testing procedures would have reduced the anxiety levels of both child and parent as they entered the diagnostic session.

Similar problems were identified when the speech-language pathologist interpreted the results of the evaluation to the parents. Apparently some speech-language pathologists presented their findings to parents in the presence of the child. In these cases, the parents indicated that it was difficult to attend to the explanation of the speech-language pathologist while trying to calm their child. Further, some parents indicated that the first interpretation should be short; detailed results could be discussed at a later time.

The language used by the speech-language pathologist also confused some of the parents. Although professionals are conversant with the jargon, they should remember that this terminology is new and unfamiliar to many of the parents. Vague directions were also given to the parents. They were instructed to work with their child at home but were sometimes not given specific directions on how much time to spend in such supportive therapy.

Another criticism offered by parents was that they were not kept informed of progress. And, even though the parents realized that a specific prognosis was impossible, they wanted some idea of the time frame for habilitation-rehabilitation so that they could make necessary arrangements. Parents also indicated that they were unprepared to deal with emotional problems in the home that resulted from the therapy program. Apparently, some nonhandicapped siblings resented the time parents spent in supportive therapy with the communicatively disordered child. Several parents, while talking with each other, found that many of them were faced with similar problems and suggested that group sessions led by the speech-language pathologist would be helpful. Finally, the parents said that they were not always given specific information regarding the termination of therapy. It is important that the parents know what behavior is normal, in terms of fluctuating maintenance and of future needs for professional assistance.

In view of these comments from parents, it seems that counseling should not be limited to the time that the child is actually being seen for evaluation and therapy, but should precede the child's initial interview. The exit interview also appears to be important.

Webster (1972) also has considered ways in which speech-language pathologists could measure the success of their parent counseling efforts. Although an open-ended type of questioning can be employed to obtain the responses of parents to counseling, Webster suggests that specific questions be studied. These included the following:

- What speech-language pathologist behaviors do parents identify as helpful to them?
- Do parents prefer group or individual counseling sessions?
- Should counseling sessions be intensive, or are less frequent meetings more helpful?
- Do parents carry out supportive therapy in the home, and what is their response to such requests?
- What information regarding communicative disorders do parents find helpful?

Hoopes and Dasovich (1972) attempted to determine the views of public school speech-language pathologists on parent counseling. Specifically, they sought to explore the logistics of counseling procedures in the school setting. A total of 76 public school speech-language pathologists responded anonymously to a 17-item questionnaire. In considering the amount of time allocated for parent conferences, the investigators found differences between speech-language pathologists working in county schools and those employed in the city. City professionals spent less time in parent counseling (0 to 1/2 hour per week) than did county speech-language pathologists (15 minutes to 1 hour per week). Further, 27 percent of the city speech-language pathologists were not involved in any parent counseling. (Note that this study predated the passage of PL 94-142.) The difference between the groups might have resulted from the amount of parental cooperation given to the professionals in the two settings. County parents seemed to be more involved in the therapeutic process than did parents residing in the city. When asked if sufficient time were allowed for parent counseling, 40 percent of professionals responded affirmatively. The majority of the city speech-language pathologists indicated that they would counsel with parents if time for such meetings were available. Many county speech-language pathologists, although they had time allocated for parent conferences, felt that more time was needed.

The survey revealed that conferences were held before, during, and after school hours, or according to parent availability. In the city, parent availability seemed to to be the determining factor; county speech-language pathologists were able to hold conferences during school hours.

The respondents were asked to list three factors that determined whether parent counseling was necessary. The severity of the communicative disorder presented by the child was considered to be the most important factor, with the need to provide or obtain information ranked second and third. The importance of parent counseling was also explored. Of the county speech-language pathologists, 59 percent ranked such conferences as "important," whereas 74 percent of those employed in the city felt parent counseling was "useful."

In summary, the logistics of parent counseling in the school setting must be considered. Hoopes and Dasovitch's survey suggested that differences exist between speech-language pathologists working in city and county systems and that these differences influence the number and nature of counseling sessions. Regardless of the frequency of parental contacts, however, the majority of the respondents agreed that such conferences were important and useful.

Parent counseling, therefore, is a topic receiving increasing attention from speech-language pathologists. At one point, the question of whether the speech-language pathologist should counsel at all was raised. But since PL 94-142 mandates that parents be included in program planning for the child and that they be informed of the results of evaluative procedures, counseling is no longer an option. In looking at the qualifications of an effective counselor, one finds that they are similar to those of the effective speech-language pathologist. This is a profession devoted to communication, and it is reasonable to assume that the speech-language pathologist can use this communicative skill as a counselor.

SUPERVISION

Speech-language pathologists have served in supervisory capacities almost since the beginning of the profession. A reference to the speech-language pathologist's responsibilities as a supervisor appeared in the *Journal of Speech and Hearing Disorders* as early as 1937 (American Speech and Hearing Association Committee on Supervision in Speech Pathology and Audiology, 1978). Although several conferences have been held to define the role and training of the supervisor, and articles regarding those subjects have appeared in professional journals, there are issues that still require resolution. Although some functions of a supervisor in various settings and at different levels of training may be essentially the same, for the purposes of this discussion, a distinction is made between the role of the supervisor of student interns in the schools and the function of the supervisor of school speech, language, and hearing programs.

Supervision of School Internship

In order to qualify for certification to work in the school setting in most states, the student must undertake student teaching or a school internship.

The amount of time spent in student teaching, the academic credit hours or clock hours required, and the way in which student interns are supervised are among the factors that vary among the training institutions and states. The Rees and Smith (1967) surveyed univeristy supervisors, master clinicians (supervising school speech-language pathologists), and former students in California in an effort to ascertain whether practices in effect at that time were poor, satisfactory, or good. Although many factors were investigated, only the opinions regarding supervision are presented here.

A questionnaire devised by the researchers was sent to 25 university supervisors, 214 master clinicians, and 293 graduates of California training programs. Of the 22 university supervisors responding, 23 percent felt that the supervision provided by them was poor. Nine university supervisors (41 percent) felt that it was satisfactory, and eight (36 percent) judged their supervision as good. The majority of the master clinicians did not concur with the opinions of university supervisors regarding the adequacy of the latter's supervision. Of the 106 responding master cliniciains, 49 percent felt that university supervision of students placed in the schools was poor. It was regarded as satisfactory by 38 clinicians, while only 16 rated university supervision as good. Of the 152 students returning the questionnaire, 32 percent (48 students) felt that supervision by university personnel was poor, 23 percent (35 students) judged it to be satisfactory, and 45 percent (69 students) rated it as good. Some discrepancies were apparent in this category, but general dissatisfaction with university supervision was expressed.

More positive feedback came in response to the question of the master clinician supervision of student interns. All of the university supervisors rated such supervision in either the satisfactory or good categories; 19 of the 23 supervisors judged it to be the latter. Of the 100 master clinician responses, only 7 percent felt that their supervision was poor. Supervision was considered satisfactory by 24 percent, and 69 percent judged it to be good. Of the 149 former students who responded to this question, only 17 students (11 percent) regarded master clinician supervision as poor. The remaining students considered supervision by the school speech-language pathologists to be satisfactory (21 percent) or good (68 percent). Based on these results, the investigators did not view this as a problem area.

A major function of the supervisor is the evaluation of the individuals for whom he or she is responsible. Rees and Smith (1967), in looking at this area of responsibility, found some inconsistencies. Although the majority of university supervisors (59 percent) felt that their evaluative procedures were good, only 32 percent of the master clinicians and 46 percent of the former students agreed. College supervisors' evaluative practices were judged poor by 9 percent of the university personnel, 33 percent of the master clinicians, and 30 percent of the graduates. The remaining respondents considered such procedures adequate.

Greater concurrence was found when the master clinicians' evaluative practices were rated. These practices were considered good by 87 percent of the university supervisors, 58 percent of the master clinicians, and 60 percent of the former students. None of the university personnel were dissatisfied with master clinician evaluative practices, and just 13 percent of the school speech-language pathologists and 16 percent of the former students judged these practices to be poor. Although this did not seem to be a particularly troublesome area, the investigators felt that revision of master clinician evaluation procedures might be considered.

The written evaluation criteria provided by the university were also analyzed. The majority of all three groups felt that the criteria were satisfactory or good, and only 6 percent of the university supervisors, 24 percent of the master clinicians, and 13 percent of the former students regarded them as poor. Again, enough dissatisfaction was expressed to warrant revision of the written evaluation criteria provided by the university.

Some districts in California provide master clinicians with written criteria for the evaluation of student speech-language pathologists. When such criteria were employed, the majority of the supervisors, master clinicians, and former students found them to be satisfactory or good. Of the 138 responses, 17 percent of the supervisors, 16 percent of the master clinicians, and 24 percent of the students regarded them as poor. These results suggested that revision of district criteria might be necessary.

With regard to supervision of student speech-language pathologists in the schools, then, Rees and Smith (1967) identified several problems. Areas requiring improvement were supervision by university personnel and evaluation procedures employed by both universities and individual school districts. The supervisory practices of master clinicians were well regarded by all three groups.

In a follow-up article, Rees and Smith (1968) reported on the results of the second part of their questionnaire. In this report, elements affecting the quality of the programs were discussed. One of the factors explored was the package of the recommended qualifications for university supervisors and master clinicians. It was agreed that the supervisor should carry university teaching assignments, hold ASHA certification, and have had experience in the public schools. The academic degree required for a university supervisor and the necessity of prior full-time clinical experiences were issues that required additional study. The qualifications of master clinicians were also explored. The respondents recommended that master clinicians have at least three years of experience, but they did not reach a consensus regarding the academic degree required or the necessity for the CCC-SP.

Supervisory practices were also investigated by Rees and Smith (1968). It was recommended that the university supervisor confer with both the student and the master clinician whenever the supervisor visited the school. Further study was required to determine the number of visits the university supervisor should make to observe each student speech-language pathologist. The respondents seemed to think that between three and six visits would be appropriate.

Regarding evaluation procedures, it was recommended that independent written evaluations of students be completed by the master clinician and the university supervisor. These evaluations should allow for both objective data and narrative judgments and should be presented orally to the student. Weekly oral evaluations of the student by the master clinician should transpire, and students should also be given the opportunity to evaluate themselves. Finally, it was recommended that students evaluate the school program in writing. No consensus was reached regarding the need for a cooperatively prepared written evaluation of the student by the master clinician and the university supervisor. Similarly, the number of required oral evaluations of the student by the university supervisor and master clinician together was not determined.

Based on the investigation of Rees and Smith, the California Conference on Standards for Supervised Experience for Speech and Hearing Specialists in Public Schools was held in 1969 (Monnin & Peters, 1977). During the three-day conference, former students, master clinicians, and university supervisors discussed various components of the public school practicum program. A set of guidelines emerged from these discussions, and these guidelines were incorporated into the training program at California State University at Los Angeles. In addition to the creation of a directed-teaching program, the functions of university supervisors and the evaluative process were considered.

The university supervisor should visit the school on a "regular" basis to observe the student speech-language pathologist. The university supervisor and the master clinician should discuss these observations; the university supervisor, student, and master clinician should also confer. When problems arise, additional supervisory visits and conferences can be scheduled. Concurrent with the student teaching experience, student speech-language pathologists are enrolled in a seminar taught by the university supervisor. Student contact and continuity in the directed-teaching program are facilitated by attendance at the seminar.

Formal evaluations of the student speech-language pathologists by the master clinicians are conducted midway and at the end of the directed-teaching experience. The university supervisor prepares a written evaluation at the end of the assignment. Since grading is on a credit–fail basis, these written evaluations are critical. Finally, students are required to assess the directed-teaching experience, and their evaluations are utilized to analyze and make necessary programmatic modifications.

Baldes, Goings, Herbold, Jeffrey, Wheeler, and Freilinger (1977) addressed the evaluation of student speech-language pathologists and concur that frequent evaluative sessions should be held. They have also devised an instrument for evaluating students that assesses the student's capabilities in identification, diagnosis, scheduling, and therapeutic management. Additionally, the student's ability to maintain appropriate relationships with other professionals and with the client and his or her family is evaluated. Baldes et al. also recommended certain experiences, including opportunities to identify, evaluate, and schedule children, as well as to plan and deliver services to them. The students should also participate in record keeping, consultation, and public relations and have some administrative experiences.

This sampling of the literature provides some idea of what supervisors involved in school practica are required to do. Ideally, the university supervisor and the responsible public school speech-language pathologist(s) should develop the goals and objectives of the school internship program cooperatively. The time frame for the experience is governed by individual state requirements and university academic calendars. Although most supervision by cooperating speech-language pathologists is quite intensive, less frequent observations are made by university personnel. Evaluations, both oral and written, should be sufficiently comprehensive to keep students informed of their progress; similarly, student evaluation of the school internship experience should allow school and university professionals to analyze the program and make necessary adjustments.

Although the foregoing information should be of interest to the reader, one specific question remains unexplored. How does one supervise the student in training? Supervision, according to *Webster's Dictionary*, is "the direction and critical evaluation of instruction, especialy in the public schools." Direction of the student teaching experience should have been established prior to or at the beginning of the program. Both the student and the supervisor should be aware of the experiences the student is to have and of the means by which appropriate opportunities will be made available. The direction of the experience, therefore, should not be difficult. Evaluating the student's performance, on the other hand, may present problems.

The competent, confident school speech-language pathologist recognizes that there are several ways of handling service delivery. Although one professional may feel more comfortable with programmed therapy, another may achieve positive results with traditional approaches. For this reason, school speech-language pathologists must not attempt to create carbon copies of themselves and must not evaluate students in terms of their ability to fit into a specific mold. Acceptance of individual therapeutic styles, then, is a prerequisite for supervisors.

An instinct for when to be directive and when to allow students to make discoveries on their own is another attribute of a good supervisor. When student experimentation is not deleterious to the children in therapy, it should be permitted. Nothing is more disheartening or confidence shattering than for the supervisor to take over a session for which the student is responsible.

Demonstration therapy is perfectly acceptable, but repossession of a session reduces the childrens' respect for the student speech-language pathologist, as well as the student's confidence in himself or herself.

A similar statement can be made about critical analysis of the student's performance. Too often the supervisor recites a litany of the student's errors and shortcomings with little attention to his or her strengths. With experienced students, self-evaluation serves a better purpose than supervisory assessment. Students should be given the opportunity to reflect on their own performances and to analyze them with the help of the supervisor. The ability to evaluate oneself is, after all, one of the ultimate objectives of training.

The supervising school speech-language pathologist must also be alert to the student's readiness to assume responsibilities. Students must be introduced to new situations and duties in a systematic and gradual manner. Some school speech-language pathologists appear to hold a "sink or swim" attitude; others seem reluctant to relinquish any responsibility. The effective supervisor is sensitive to the student's readiness and delegates appropriate responsibilities in a carefully planned sequence.

Obviously, these observations do not begin to answer the question, "How does one supervise the student in training?" Supervision is an art, just as counseling parents or executing therapy are. Acceptance of and respect for the student along with a commitment to training students for public school work are important. In the author's experience with many supervising speech-language pathologists, however, the traits discussed above seem to separate the effective supervisors from those with lesser abilities.

Supervision of School Speech, Language, and Hearing Programs

Interest in the supervision of professionals employed in the schools has increased in the past decade. The state of Indiana pioneered in the study of supervision in the school setting by holding conferences in 1966 and 1969 (Anderson, 1970). In 1970, state and local supervisors as well as university personnel involved in supervision convened at Indiana University to discuss the supervision of school speech, language, and hearing programs. The following material is extracted from notes from that conference (as reported in Anderson, 1970).

During a panel discussion, the training of supervisors of school speech, language, and hearing programs was discussed. The total function of a supervisor may be broken down into those activities that are supervisory and those that require administrative skills. Supervisors, according to participant Peters, should be competent speech-language pathologists; further, some of the supervisor's clinical experience should be in the school setting. Training, however, is necessary to transform a skilled clinician into a competent supervisor. Peters suggests that this training should occur at the post-master's level after the speech-language pathologist has had some experience. Such training should include exposure to theories and methods involved in the supervisory process. Supervisory experience in a practicum setting should supplement the course work. A second area to be considered in training the supervisor is that of human interaction. Peters feels that many problems encountered by supervisors relate to their inability to relate to supervisees, "Whether we use sensitivity groups, encounter groups, therapy groups, individual counseling or whatever, it is important that we have a way to develop the ability of supervisors to understand themselves and others and to learn to interact effectively with others" (Anderson, 1970, p. 131). A third area of training deals with clinical research skills; according to Peters, there should be less emphasis in this area.

Regarding administrative functions, supervisors should understand and be competent in such areas as budget preparation and program management. Peters suggests that this competence might result from participation in courses dealing with organizational theory, business management, and educational administration.

Although Peters' remarks were conceptual in nature, Wood described the training procedures utilized at the University of Texas for the preparation of supervisors. Advanced graduate students with at least 200 clinical clock hours may participate in a graduate course in supervision, while supervising a team of student speech-language pathologists. The student supervisors are supervised by a staff member. The thrusts of all course work and supervisor experiences are in three areas: administration, instruction, and clinical supervision. In the administrative area, students discuss such topics as personnel management, relations with the public, and working conditions. Listening skills, behavioral observation and description, and methods of offering criticism are among the topics considered in "instruction." The final area of training is the application of supervisory or administrative skills in a practicum setting. Although Peters' concept of a training process for supervisors and the in-place program described by Wood are similar, the time at which students and/or professionals would receive such training differs. Wood points out, however, that some professional employment as a speech-language pathologist should precede advancement to a supervisory position.

Prior to the 1970 Indiana conference, a survey was conducted to ascertain the status of supervision in school programs for communicatively disordered children (Anderson, 1972). Questionnaires were mailed to 527 individuals thought to be supervisors of speech, language, and hearing programs. A total of 211 questionnaires were returned by 118 part-time and 93 full-time supervisors.

The respondents, who were variously titled "supervisor," "coordinator," or "director," typically were individuals with master's degrees, although some had bachelor's degrees, and a small percentage held doctorates. Among the respondents, 27 percent of the full-time and 22 percent of the part-time supervisors reported that they had had course work in supervision; only 20 individuals had had a specific course in the supervision of speech and hearing programs. The overwhelming majority of the respondents had had public school experience, ranging from 1 to 26 years.

Respondents were asked not only to provide descriptive information about themselves but to identify the three biggest problems they had encountered as supervisors. Full-time supervisors varied in their responses; the professional inadequacies of the school speech-language pathologists and the need for additional personnel headed the list. Part-time supervisors identified insufficient time to execute their responsibilities as the most significant problem.

When asked whether special training for supervisor positions was necessary, 92 percent of the full-time and 81 percent of the part-time supervisors answered affirmatively. According to the respondents, the training should include information related to supervisory techniques, methods of evaluation, counseling and interviewing strategies, and in-service training. Business management material should be included, as should content information in speech-language pathology and audiology. Additionally. supervisors should obtain training in school administration.

Finally, the respondents were asked to estimate the amount of time consumed each week by various activities. Observation of school speech-language pathologists, staff meetings, program development activities, and diagnostic sessions occupied a large percentage of both the full-time and part-time supervisors' week. Other activities, including in-service training and correspondence, required considerable attention.

The results of this survey revealed that the preparation of supervisors is inconsistent and that supervisors of school speech, language, and hearing programs encounter a diversity of problems. It is apparent that the training of such professionals should be more specialized and should include information on program management as well as supervisory techniques.

Anderson (1974) identified four responsibilities that the profession must assume with regard to the supervision of school programs for the communicatively disordered. First, it is necessary to persuade school administrators of the need for supervisors. Next, the role of such supervisors must be defined; components of the supervisory process and the competencies of supervisor must also be identified. Finally, the profession should establish training programs for supervisors.

According to Anderson, the need for program supervisors becomes apparent if three factors are considered. Initially, when staff reductions occur, appropriate utilization of the remaining professionals is imperative. A competent supervisor can direct and coordinate this effort. Additionally, accountability trends in the schools demand that supervisors with administrative and

supervisory skills be employed to manage program development and evaluation services. Finally, the mandate of education for all handicapped children
requires that a more comprehensive continuum of services be provided to
these students. This type of programming requires administrative skills that
can only be found in a competent supervisor.

Regarding the role of the school supervisor, little specificity is evident.
As indicated by others, both administrative and supervisory skills are
necessary; in addition the supervisor should be able to serve in a leadership
capacity. Generally, however, all activities of the supervisor should be
directed toward insuring that competent services are delivered to communicatively disordered children.

The competencies of effective supervisors must be identified. According
to Anderson (1974), "The profession as a whole should begin to identify
those competencies needed by all supervisors of the clinical process and those
competencies needed in specific job environments" (p. 9). Definition of these
competencies will assist training programs in devising curricula to prepare
supervisors for school speech, language, and hearing programs.

In discussing the training of supervisors, Anderson suggests that the profession should not be reactionary to state certification boards. Instead, university programs should develop a body of course work that will include information on supervision, business management, advanced material in speech-
language pathology, educational administration, and research techniques.
Practicum experiences should also be provided. According to Anderson (1974),
the professional faces a challenge with regard to the issue of supervision. "It remains to be seen whether we will accept that challenge" (p. 10).

ASHA responded to the need to establish guidelines for school programs
with the publication of *Standards and Guidelines for Comprehensive
Language, Speech, and Hearing Programs in the Schools* (American Speech
and Hearing Association, 1973–1974). Included in the manual were recommendations for program supervisors and five specific guidelines.

First, it was recommended that a supervisor be provided for each school
speech, language, and hearing program. A part-time supervisor may serve
when the total staff consists of fewer than 10 speech-language pathologists. A
staff containing 10 to 29 members should have a full-time supervisor, and one
additional supervisor should be provided for every 15 staff members over 29.
Additionally, programs with more than 20 to 30 staff members should have a
full-time administrator as well as a full-time supervisor.

It was recommended that the frequency and nature of supervision should
depend on the qualifications and capabilities of the staff members being supervised. Specifically, the manual provides that (1) master's-level professionals in
their initial year of employment should be supervised at least 15 percent of the
time they are involved in service delivery, and (2) bachelor's-level staff in their
first year must be directly supervised 20 percent of their service deliver time;

thereafter, 15 percent of the student contact time must be observed.

Program management guidelines were also provided. The manual recommends that the supervisor should

- Develop program goals and objectives
- Develop data collection systems
- Participate in recruitment, employment, and dismissal of professional and subprofessional staff
- Deploy staff members according to their abilities and program needs
- Determine guidelines for case identification, selection, scheduling, and disposition
- Secure functional and appropriate physical facilities for staff members and the program
- Participate in increasing public awareness of services provided by the program
- Prepare budgets and request materials and equipment for the staff
- Coordinate school practicum experiences for university students in training
- Observe and assess staff and paraprofessionals

The supervisor should also play a consultative role by serving as a resource person to the staff and paraprofessionals, as well as in parent counseling. The improvement of direct services is one of the supervisor's responsibilities in this area, as is participation in educational curricular development.

Finally, the supervisor must participate in program development and assessment. In this role, the supervisor may initiate in-service training programs, work with parents, create innovative service delivery strategies, and develop grant proposals.

The duties of the supervisor according to the ASHA guidelines, therefore, are extremely diverse. Certainly training is required to execute these numerous responsibilities with competence, and more than efficiency as a speech-language pathologist is required for the role of supervisor.

The American Speech and Hearing Association Committee on Supervision in Speech Pathology and Audiology (1978) has identified and defined nine issues that are related to supervision and that are of concern to members of the profession. The first of these issues is the need for data validating the effectiveness of supervision. According to the Committee report, "We have no data to indicate that supervision makes a difference in the effectiveness of clinicians at any level of training or in the employment setting" (American Speech and Hearing Association Committee on Supervision in Speech Pathology and Audiology, 1978, p. 480). Furthermore, in the area of supervision limited research is being conducted that might provide the necessary information. Research that has been done lacks a publication outlet. This need is critical, since many other issues involved in supervision are related to the lack of validating information.

A second need, one that has been discussed previously, is for definition of the supervisor's role. The Committee reported that too frequently supervisors begin to function in that role without preparation for it or a specific definition of their responsibilities. Guidelines in this area are imperative.

Although there appears to be a need for additional supervisors, the Committee found this need difficult to support with hard data. Regarding supervision in the schools, it is estimated that there is one supervisor to every 38 speech-language pathologists rather than the one to 10 ratio recommended in the ASHA Guidelines. Dublinske (cited in American Speech and Hearing Association Committee on Supervision in Speech Pathology and Audiology, 1978) estimated that to meet those recommendations, over 1900 supervisors should be employed. Finally, there is evidence that even when supervisors are employed, they may not be qualified to oversee staff activities. Again, information in this area is incomplete, but limited evidence suggests that additional supervisors are needed.

Other needs identified by the Committee were the need for improvement in the quality of supervisors and the need for standards. For an individual to supervise in the schools, it is recommended that he or she have a CCC-SP, have had at least three years of experience in the schools, and be certified in the state of employment. Other competencies or characteristics required for effective supervision remain unclear.

The need for training of supervisors was identified by the Committee. Citing the results of studies that indicated that many supervisors have received little or no training before assuming supervisory positions, a distinct deficit was noted. Similarly, it was determined that many university training programs do not offer appropriate course work in this area. Supervisors responding to various surveys also indicated a need for training. It may easily be concluded, therefore, that additional training opportunities for supervisors must be provided.

As this review of the literature suggests, the role of the speech-language pathologist as a supervisor of school speech, language, and hearing programs is somewhat unfocused. The competencies, characteristics, training, and specific responsibilities require additional study by professionals so that guidelines may be established.

REFERENCES

Ainsworth, S. The speech clinician in public schools: "participant" or "separatist"? *Asha,* 1964, *7,* 495–503.

Albritton, T. The school clinician and ASHA in the seventies. *Language, Speech, and Hearing Services in Schools,* 1970, *2,* 3–6.

American Speech and Hearing Association Committee on Definitions of Public School Speech and Hearing Services. Services and functions of speech and hearing specialists in public schools. *Asha,* 1962, *4,* 99–100.

American Speech and Hearing Association Committee on Speech and Hearing Services in the Public Schools. The speech clinician's role in the public school. *Asha,* 1964, *6,* 189–191.

American Speech and Hearing Association Committee on Supervision in Speech Pathology and Audiology. Current status of supervision of speech-language pathology and audiology. *Asha,* 1978, *20,* 478–486.

American Speech and Hearing Association. *Standards and guidelines for comprehensive language, speech and hearing programs in the schools.* Washington, D.C., 1973–1974.

Anderson, J. L. (Ed.). *Conference on supervision of speech and hearing programs in the schools.* Bloomington: Indiana University Press, 1970.

Anderson, J. L. Status of supervision of speech, hearing and language programs in the schools. *Language, Speech, and Hearing Services in Schools,* 1972, *3,* 12–22.

Anderson, J. L. Supervision of school speech, hearing and language programs—an emerging role. *Asha,* 1974, *16,* 7–10.

Baldes, R. A., Goings, R., Herbold, D. D., Jeffrey, R., Wheeler, G., & Freilinger, J. J. Supervision of student speech clinicians. *Language, Speech, and Hearing Services in Schools,* 1977, *8,* 76–84.

Black, M. *Speech correction in the schools.* Englewood Cliffs: Prentice-Hall, 1964.

Bown, J. C. The expanding responsibilities of the speech and hearing clinician in the public schools. *Journal of Speech and Hearing Disorders,* 1971, *36,* 538–542.

Dublinske, S. New opportunities for speech-language pathologists and audiologists, *Asha,* 1979, *21,* 998–1002.

Eisenstadt, A. A. Weakness in clinical procedures—A parental evaluation. *Asha,* 1972, *14,* 7–9.

Emerick, L. *The parent interview.* Danville: The Interstate Printers & Publishers, Inc., 1969.

Falck, V. T. Communication skills—Translating theory into practice. *Teaching Exceptional Children,* 1978, *10,* 74–77.

Flynn, P. T. Effective clinical interviewing. *Language, Speech, and Hearing Services in Schools,* 1978, *9,* 265–271.

Hoopes, M., & Dasovich, M. O. Parent counseling: A survey of use by the public school speech clinician. *Journal of the Missouri Speech and Hearing Assocation,* 1972, *5,* 9–13.

Monnin, L. M., & Peters, K. M. Problem solving supervised experiences in the schools. *Language, Speech and Hearing Services in Schools,* 1977, *8,* 99–106.

Powers, M. H. What makes an effective public school speech therapist. *Journal of Speech and Hearing Disorders.* 1956, *21,* 461–467.

Rees, M., & Smith, G. Supervised school experience for student clinicians. *Asha,* 1967, *9,* 251–256.

Rees, M., & Smith, G. L. Some recommendations for supervised school experience for student clinicians. *Asha,* 1968, *10,* 93–103.

Stewart, J. C. *Counseling parents of exceptional children.* Columbus: Charles E. Merrill Publishing Company, 1978.

Van Hattum, R. J. *Clinical speech in the schools.* Springfield: Charles C Thomas, 1969.

Van Hattum, R. J. Services of the speech clinician in schools: Progress and prospects. *Asha,* 1976, *18,* 59–63.

Van Hattum, R. J. The defensive speech clinicians in the schools. *Journal of Speech and Hearing Disorders,* 1966, *31,* 234–240.

Weaver, J. B. An investigation of attitudes of speech clinicians in the public schools. *Asha,* 1968, *10,* 319–322.

Webster, E. J. Parent counseling by speech pathologists and audiologists. *Journal of Speech and Hearing Disorders,* 1966, *31,* 331–340.

Webster, E. J. Procedures for group parent counseling in speech pathology and audiology. *Journal of Speech and Hearing Disorders,* 1968, *33,* 127–131.

Webster, E. J. Questions regarding parental responses to parent counseling. *Language, Speech and Hearing Services in Schools,* 1972, *3,* 47–50.

Webster, E. J., & Cole, B. M. Effective leadership of parent discussion groups. *Language, Speech, and Hearing Services in Schools,* 1979, *10,* 72–80.

9

Supportive Personnel

Carefully supervised, well planned, with clearly defined goals and responsibilities, the communication aide program can enhance public school speech therapy and provide opportunities to significantly expand, without diluting, the quality of services of the speech clinician serving the school. (Braunstein, 1972, pp. 34–35).

In recent years, the utilization of paraprofessionals in a variety of disciplines has increased. The medical, social, and educational fields have recognized that employing supportive personnel can improve the quality of service delivery, as well as the quantity of such services. Speech-language pathologists are now dealing with the issue of paraprofessionals, and many are experimenting with the utilization of both paid and/or volunterer supportive personnel. Although many questions remain to be answered, it is apparent that parents, students at the preprofessional level of training in speech-pathology, high school graduates, and retrained paraprofessionals have been and are being used to provide specific services to speech and language impaired children and adolescents.

PARENTS AS SUPPORTIVE PERSONNEL

It is a recognized fact that the success of therapeutic services delivered to children in schools and clinics depends to some degree on the involvement of parents. Neither the traditional service delivery schedule nor intensive cycle scheduling allows sufficient time for the monitoring necessary to modify

169

speech and language patterns efficiently. Even more intensive programs, such as those available in self-contained or resource rooms, fail to provide the before and after school, weekend, and vacation stimulation and instruction that may be necessary. For years, speech-language pathologists have attempted to involve parents in the therapeutic process. These attempts were often sporadic and unorganized. Even today, the main communication between parents and speech-language pathologists may take place during the required IEP conferences and in notes attached to the child's speech book. It is encouraging that speech-language pathologists are defining the role of the parent in the habilitative process and implementing programs in which the parents can participate more vigorously.

Parental Involvement
with Multiply Handicapped Children

Early reports of the utilization of parents, specifically the mother, came in 1948. Lillywhite (1948) addressed the issue of the habilitation of severely handicapped children including those with cerebral palsy, aphasia, and delayed speech. Although his specific concern was with supplementing work done in a university speech clinic, the confidence that Lillywhite placed in mothers to implement language training programs is revealing. The original participant was the self-trained mother of a brain injured child. Having been told that there was no hope for her son and that he should be institutionalized, this mother, a speech major in college, successfully undertook his habilitation. Later employed by the college, the mother then trained other mothers to deal with their aphasic children. Although success was reported in most instances, one failure was identified. The unsuccessful mother was hearing impaired and apparently suffered from severe guilt regarding her son. Lillywhite suggests that other factors may contraindicate the effective training of mothers; these include poor health, disinterest in the program, outside employment, or ininadequate intelligence. In general, the experiences reported by Lillywhite indicate that mothers can be used effectively. He suggests that appropriate reading material be assigned to supplement training sessions. Although time is required to train and supervise mothers, Lillywhite suggests that the time is well invested.

Parental Involvement with Children
with Articulatory Disorders

Sommers, Schilling, Paul, Copetas, Bowser, and McClintock (1959) investigated the training of parents of children with functional articulatory disorders. The subjects were 72 children enrolled in two speech clinics; the experimental and control groups each consisted of 36 children. The functional nature of the articulatory defects was established after evaluating intelligence, hearing, articulation, and the structure and functioning of the speech mechanism. The children were then assigned to one of two groups; the experimental and control groups were matched according to sex, intelligence, number of articulatory errors, and frequency of clinic attendance.

Prior to implementation of therapy, extensive pretesting of articulation was done and therapist reliability was established. The therapy itself consisted of four consecutive one-hour group sessions each week for three and one-half weeks. In general, therapeutic procedures were based on Van Riper's traditional methods. Weekly meetings of the six participating speech-language pathologists were held to assure the uniformity of therapy techniques. Although homogeneity in direct therapy was stressed, the participation of parents of the two groups differed. Parents of control group children were invited to attend discussion groups; experimental group parents were told that attendance at daily meetings was necessary. While the children attended therapy, the parents participated in 30-minute lecture-discussion sessions. Topics included speech development and communicative disorders but stressed the nature of therapy and procedures that could be employed at home to supplement therapy. Following the daily discussion group meetings, experimental group parents observed therapy. Opportunities for discussion of the therapy sessions with the speech-language pathologist were available, and specific suggestions were made for work at home. Control group parents, on the other hand, did not observe therapy, and they received no instruction on ways to deal with the child at home. Although each child had a speech book, specific assignments were not explained to the control group parents. Three group meetings were held between the speech-language pathologist and the control group parents but these were brief and general.

The results of the study suggest that concurrent training of children and their parents may facilitate the modification of articulatory disorders. Improvement of substitution errors was particularly apparent in the experimental group, although little change in distortion or omission errors was noted in either group. Although overwhelming differences between the experimental and control groups were not apparent, the authors suggest that a longer period of therapy and training might have produced more significant changes. They caution that the approach involved in the study was carefully devised and that similar results might not be obtained with a more anxiety-producing program.

In an attempt to decrease the number of children entering school with functional articulatory errors, Tufts and Holliday (1959) designed a program to train parents whose preschoolers exhibited misarticulations. The researchers selected 43 preschool children with normal hearing and intelligence who did not evidence abnormal functioning of the speech mechanism. All were judged to have moderate articulatory defects. Of these children, 30 were assigned to one of three groups. Group A received no speech therapy, Group B received assistance from a speech-language pathologist, and Group C received help from their parents. Following a pretherapy assessment of articulatory skills (Trial I), the children participated in a seven-month program. Although the parents of Group A children were told about the study and assured that necessary therapy would be provided to their children at its conclusion, they were instructed not to attempt any remedial procedures. Group B children were involved in 46 direct therapy sessions with a speech-language pathologist. Traditional group therapy procedures were employed. Group C children were instructed by their mothers who were also meeting with the speech-language pathologist for one hour each week. At no time did the professional see the 10 Group C children; instead the speech-language pathologist advised the mothers on methods of correcting articulatory errors, and the latter implemented these suggestions.

The results of this study verify the importance of early intervention with children with articulatory disorders. Both Group B and C children showed improvement when reevaluated (Trial II) after the seven-month program. No change in articulatory skills was seen in Group A children, nor was there a significant difference between Group B and Group C children. The latter finding indicates that trained parents are as effective as speech-language pathologists in modifying the errors of children with moderate disorders. The authors suggest that school speech-language pathologists consider parental training as a means of reducing the number of children entering school with articulatory disturbances.

In an expansion of earlier studies, Sommers (1962) investigated factors related to the effectiveness of mothers in the therapeutic process. Using trained and untrained mothers of "slow" and normal children with articulatory disorders, he found that trained mothers were more effective than those without similar training. Further, children of normal intelligence made more progress than those children considered to be "slow learners." In examining maternal attitudes and effectiveness in therapy, Sommers, Furlong, Rhodes, Fichter, Bowser, Copetas, and Saunders (1964) found little interaction between maternal attitude and training. Mothers with both healthy and unhealthy attitudes, as determined by results of the Parental Attitude Research Instrument, benefited equally from the training procedure. However, children whose mothers were judged to be healthy made more improvement in articulatory skills than those with "unhealthy" mothers. Finally, the children with trained mothers once again made significantly more progress than those with untrained mothers.

Carrier (1970) devised an articulation program to be administered by mothers in the home. The six-lesson program had an operant design and was based on the *stimulus shift* concept. The 20 subjects on whom the program was tested ranged in age from 4 to 7 years; the subjects were assigned to two groups, matched in terms of age and articulatory errors. Mothers of the experimental group were trained to use the articulation program, whereas control group mothers were merely instructed to model the correct sound when their children made errors. Original instruction in the correct production of target phonemes was provided by a speech-language pathologist.

Following completion of the study, it was found that mothers were able to execute the program effectively and that children receiving programmed home training improved significantly when compared to children who received random modeling. These results reinforce the efficacy of employing mothers as supportive personnel, especially when the program is well organized and provides specific instructions.

Fudula, England, and Ganoung (1972) addressed one issue raised by speech-language pathologists as they consider the use of parent aides, that of training time. Most school personnel do not have the luxury of time allocated to work with parents; instead, the greater portion of each day is spent in direct contact with children presenting communicative disorders. In order to alleviate that problem, the possibility that parental observation of therapy might serve as a training procedure was explored.

Participants in the study were 92 children with functional articulatory disorders and their parents. All of the children had normal hearing and were of low, average, or above-average intelligence. Random assignment of the 92 children was to Group I, Group II-A, or Group II-B; the distribution of intelligence within each group was similar. Group I parents were asked not to observe therapy sessions but to work with their children five minutes per day if assignments were sent home. The speech-language pathologist maintained contact with the parents via telephone or written communication. Group II-A contained 23 children; their parents observed therapy once per month (one out of every four sessions). Group II-B parents attended each weekly session and later participated in therapy sessions.

Posttesting after one semester of therapy revealed that children in Group II made almost twice as much improvement as the children assigned to Group I. No significant differences were found between Groups II-A and II-B. Subjective reports from teachers and principals indicated that the attitudes of the parents involved in Group II improved also. Fudula and co-workers acknowledged some problems in the logistics of the program but were optimistic regarding its effectiveness in the school setting.

Wing and Heimgartner (1973) investigated the efficacy of utilizing parents in the carry-over phase of articulation therapy. Additionally, the authors sought to develop transfer procedures that were sequenced, measureable, and expeditious. In sequencing the steps, five carry-over levels, each having specific objectives, were outlined. Parents were to execute the program in order to expedite habilitative efforts. It was also felt that a program carried out in the home would be less artificial than one limited to the speech room environment.

Parents received instruction regarding the program and were taught to identify and record correct and incorrect responses. In addition, they learned how to maintain data for each session. Children also participated in the 30 to 40-minute training session so that the parents could practice listening, evaluating, and recording a speech sample. Following the training session, only telephone contact between the parents and the school speech-language pathologist was maintained.

The six subjects involved in the pilot study completed the program in an average of 40 10-minute home sessions. After three months had elapsed, carry-over into other speaking environments was regarded as good by the speech-language pathologist, teachers, and the parents. Additional children with whom the program was implemented demonstrated equally good transfer of newly acquired articulatory skills.

The investigators were pleased with the results of their program. Not only was the program successful in completing the transfer process quickly, it also released professionals to work with children presenting more complex communicative disorders. The specificity of the steps, the establishment of realistic objectives, and the maintenance of daily records of sessions were felt to contribute to the program's success.

Parental Involvement in Behavior Management

Carpenter and Augustine (1973) instructed the mothers of four children with communicative disorders in behavior management techniques. After a two-day workshop, the mothers were given lesson plans to be carried out with their children at home. Thereafter, the mothers maintained contact with the speech-language pathologist by mail and telephone. Three of the four children made positive gains during the next few months; although the fourth mother reported progress, an assessment of the child failed to confirm such improvement. The authors concluded that a similar approach might be effective in the absence of speech-language pathology services or when daily therapy is needed.

Parental Involvement with Language Disorders

In 1972, Bush and Bonachea (1973) initiated the Parents' Advice on Language, or PAL, program. Assuming that the language disordered child needs frequent stimulation in a variety of environments, parents were enlisted as supportive personnel. Initially, language specialists made home visits to parents of first and second grade children with deficiencies in receptive or expressive language. Later, the parents were invited to participate in a home language program.

Those parents who chose to join in the program attended weekly meetings to discuss their experiences and problems. Semi-instructional programs were presented at these metings, and on occasion, there were guest speakers. Parents also exchanged ideas and prepared materials for language stimulation in the home. Specific instructions for home projects and experiences were also presented to the parents, and they were instructed in the use of corrective feedback. Weekly data charts were kept by parents to record the results of the parent–child projects.

The success of the PAL program led to its expansion to other grade levels and schools within the district. In addition to home projects, the PAL II program included more frequent field trips and neighborhood activities. The authors attributed the success of the PAL programs to several factors. Among them was the attitude of the speech-language pathologist toward the parents; the latter were treated with respect, and their advice was given careful consideration in the program. Additionally, the fact that home projects were inexpensive and based on ordinary family and home activities seemed to contribute to the parents' enthusiasm for the program.

MacDonald, Blott, Gordon, Spiegel, and Hartmann (1974) initiated a multipurpose investigation of language programming for preschool, language delayed children. One of the questions asked was whether parents could be taught to execute the language program so as to effect transfer into the home environment. Six Down's syndrome children and their families participated in the study, three as experimental subjects and three as controls. The Environmental Language Intervention Strategy was employed.

Phase I of the two-phase, five-month experimental program involved a seven-week training program at the Nisonger Center. The speech-language pathologists and the mothers were involved in sessions twice weekly at the Center, while the mothers executed daily training at home. During Phase II, the mothers worked at home with the children and met monthly with the professional language trainers. Improvement noted during Phase I of the program continued to occur during the second phase when the mothers alone served as language trainers. MacDonald et al. concluded that parents could indeed be taught to execute a successful home language program successfully.

This sampling of research involving parents as supportive personnel suggests that they can play significant roles in the modification of their children's communicative problems. Those programs which provide specific instructions appear to lend themselves particularly well to execution by parents.

OTHER SUPPORTIVE PERSONNEL

Preprofessional Students as Supportive Personnel

The utilization of preprofessional students in training as supportive personnel has been examined in the past and continues to receive consideration. In some cases, a paucity of trained professionals prompts school districts to opt for utilization of uncertified persons. This need may be complimented by a university's need to provide training facilities for its students. Such was the case in Mississippi when student speech and hearing "teams" were deployed to the public schools (Wingo, 1970). In this program, four undergraduates and one graduate student constituted a team. The students were assigned to centrally located public schools where they worked with communicatively disordered children. "Mild" problems were handled by undergraduates, while children with more complex communicative disorders wre the responsibility of the graduate student. A staff member from the university provided one-third-time supervision. Wingo, in analyzing the "team" program, emphasized its positive aspects. He stated that university students were exposed to a variety of children presenting diverse communicative disorders; such exposure was impossible in the university setting alone. Further, school children received services that had not been provided previously. Finally, it should be added that these services were provided at no apparent cost to the schools.

In Iowa, a program designed to provide introductory clinical training to preprofessional speech-language pathology students was instituted (Hall & Knutson, 1978). Eighteen students, having completed coursework in the basic communication areas and a course in articulatory disorders, were assigned to work with 10 children with isolated articulatory errors. All of the experimental children had been taught to produce the target phoneme in isolation by the supervising speech-language pathologist. Following a two-part orientation session during which the communication aides were introduced to the school setting and had their roles defined, they began the three-month program. Each of the 10 children was seen twice weekly for 30-minute sessions; in some cases, a single aide serviced the same child on both days whereas in others, the child had two different aides. Early in the program, session plans were devised by the school speech-language pathologist. Later, the aides wrote their own plans. Supervision and consultation were provided by the school speech-language pathologist.

Positive results accrued from the program. As was true in the Mississippi program, the researchers mentioned access to the school setting as being beneficial to the preprofessional students. At the same time, the public school children received services that might not have been available to them otherwise.

Nonprofessionals as Supportive Personnel

In a frequently cited article, Alpiner, Ogden, and Wiggins (1970) described the utilization of speech aides in a pilot study conducted in Denver, Colorado. The investigators selected 10 speech aides who met 4 minimum requirements: each was at least 18 years of age, had a high school diploma, wanted to work with children, and had access to transportation. A three-week training program preceded the entrance of the speech aides into the school setting. Instructed by university and school personnel, the aides were introduced to such topics as the organization of public schools, the speech-language pathologist's role in the schools, the speech and hearing mechanism, and the nature of communicative disorders. Orientation was also provided to the 14 public school speech-language pathologists who agreed to supervise the speech aides.

At the conclusion of the project, questionnaires were completed by the aides and the supervising speech-language pathologists. The results of the survey showed that the majority of the speech aides' time was spent in assisting with articulation therapy (51 percent), and that considerable time was spent in clerical activities (29 percent). Other responsibilities listed in descending order of frequency were assisting in language therapy (14 percent), in hearing therapy (4 percent) and in rate and rhythm therapy (one percent). The aides did not participate in voice therapy. Of the 14 supervising speech-language pathologists, 11 expressed interest in continuing to work with aides. Only 2 of the professionals did not want assistants and indicated that aides should not be imposed on the schools by the state. The majority (11) of speech-language pathologists felt that the individual professional should have the right to determine whether an aide would be useful.

In addition to the four minimum requirements mentioned, it was suggested that aides should have clerical experience, two years of college, and/or university training in speech-language pathology. Although half of the supervising speech-language pathologists felt that the three-week training session was adequate, several recommended that greater familiarity with equipment and experience with specific therapeutic techniques would be helpful. Generally, the attitudes of both the aides and the speech-language pathologists toward the project were positive. It was suggested, however, that guidelines be formulated regarding supportive personnel so that the professional status of school speech-language pathologists could be maintained.

Retrained aides have also been used in speech-language therapy. Guess, Smith, and Ensminger (1971) reported on training two former psychiatric aides to serve as language developmentalists in an institution for mentally retarded children. During a one-month training period, the aides completed assigned readings and participated in informal discussions with the project director, a speech-language pathologist. The reading-discussion topics included the role of the language developmentalist, operant conditioning, communicative development of the mentally retarded, and exposure to teaching techniques and materials. Throughout the two-year duration of the study, the language developmentalists met with the project director daily to review the program and to discuss problems or programmatic modificaitons. In discussing the results of the project, Guess et al. cited the success of the retrained language developmentalists as significant. They expressed confidence that nonprofessionals, working under the supervision of speech-language pathologists, can be trained to facilitate the language acquisition of mentally retarded children.

Gray and Barker (1977) compared the performance of aides and speech-language patholologists in executing an articulation program. The researchers trained 10 teacher aides and 9 speech-language pathologists to use the Monterey Articulation Program. After attaining proficiency with this tool, the aides and speech-language pathologists administered the program to 84 selected students. Posttest results indicated that the aides were as successful as the speech-language pathologists in obtaining positive results. The authors concluded that communication aides can effectively deliver specific services to children with articulatory disorders.

In Minnesota, paraprofessionals were trained to screen and provide services to children eight years or older presenting lateral or frontal sibilant distortions or distorted /r/ (Strong, 1972). Nine women with normal communicative abilities and speech sound discrimination were employed as technicians. All had completed high school and had plans to stay in the geographic area.

During the 16-week training program, the technicians received both academic instruction and practicum experience. Among the areas covered in the academic sequence were discrimination training and information regarding the acquisition and management of /r/ and the sibilants. Although the technicians were not trained to deal with children with vocal, rhythmic, or linguistic disorders, they were able to recognize those problems that required speech-language pathologist intervention.

After being evaluated by a speech-language pathologist, children were seen for remediation by the technicians, who employed programmed approaches. All technicians were supervised by speech-language pathologists who had received instruction in the supervisory process. Of the 117 students involved in the pilot project, 89.3 percent were dismissed from therapy; the time required to reach dismissal criterion was from three to 31 hours and the mean was 10.5 hours.

The author suggested that properly trained and supervised technicians were valuable in service delivery programs. Because of the technicians' work with children with articulatory disorders, speech-language pathologists were able to carry case loads of from 12 to 16 children. The time spent with each child was dictated by his or her needs rather than by the time available.

Braunstein (1972) reported on the utilization of communication aides with language disordered children. Facing an unmanageable case load, she developed a program designed to train an aide to conduct activities Braunstein had planned, to record progress, to report on student behavior, and to taperecord group language sessions. In addition, the aide was to confer with the speech-language pathologist, take part in in-service training, and assist the professional in preparing instructional materials. The communication aide was not to confer with parents or teachers, initiate any teaching activities, or make diagnostic or clinical judgments.

Candidates for the communication aide position had educations that varied from a high school diploma to two years of university education. In addition to displaying desirable personal characteristics, the selected aide had to commit herself to the program for a two-year period.

Initially, the aide observed the speech-language pathologist execute language therapy. After these observations, the speech-language pathologist and the aide discussed session content and outcomes. Later discussion included such topics as normal language acquisition and behavior modification, as well as the importance of observation and accurate reporting. The aide also met with other professionals and attended appropriate in-service training sessions. According to Braunstein, between 35 and 40 hours were consumed by this phase of training.

In the next training phase, the aide assumed responsibility for the language groups while the speech-language pathologist observed. Postsession discussions between the aide and the professional were facilitated by analysis of audio and videotapes of therapy. The aide was able to assume independent responsibility for sessions after 25 to 30 hours of directly supervised therapy management.

The project produced positive results, evidenced by the childrens' progress. All concerned, including teachers and parents, were enthusiastic about the communication-aide concept and supported continuation of the program. According to the author, the carefully planned and supervised utilization of a communication aide enhanced the total intervention program without neutralizing the quality of services.

Galloway and Blue (1975) described the use of paraprofessionals in executing a program for children with mild to moderate articulatory disorders. This project covered a three-year period during which each of the 39 paraprofessionals worked with an average of 9 students. The case load varied from 2 to 15 children, and some group work supplemented individual instruction.

Regarding preparation, all paraprofessionals underwent a 70-hour training program prior to the beginning of the first school year. Additional training was required during the summer, as were 45 hours of in-service training during the school year. This training focused on the use of programmed materials and procedures employed in the remedial process. All training and supervision were done by certified speech-language pathologists.

In discussing the success of this program, Galloway and Blue pointed out that the utilization of paraprofessionals permitted the provision of speech services to children who would not otherwise have received them. Secondly, the speech-language pathologist was able to reduce his or her case load while expanding services to children previously underserved. Moreover, test-retest results showed that the paraprofessionals had been successful in modifying the articulatory errors of the children they serviced. The authors, like others who have been involved in programs employing paraprofessionals, indicated that properly trained and supervised supportive personnel contribute positively to the total service delivery program.

The expansion of services to communicatively disordered children in the Los Angeles Unified School District was the purpose of a supportive personnel program instituted during the 1972–1973 school year (Scalero & Eskenazi, 1976). Both volunteers and paid aides were trained to work with children presenting articulatory and linguistic disorders. Following guidelines established by ASHA, aides were expected to present specific personal qualifications. Additionally, they were evaluated in terms of their communicative abilities, both oral and written, and their skill in learning to use relevant pieces of equipment. Entrance qualifications included being a high school graduate, having completed the training course satisfactorily, and the possession of a driver's license. Typing skill was considered desirable.

Both general and specific duties were assigned to the volunteers and aides. General responsibilities included assisting the speech-language pathologist in improving the articulatory and linguistic skills of the children, preparing instructional materials, and performing clerical duties. Specific duties involved administration of articulation and language programs and maintenance of accurate pupil performance records. Limitations were also placed on the paraprofessionals' participation in the therapeutic process.

Before the aides were assigned to schools, they received 70 hours of preservice training. The paraprofessionals were given general information concerning communicative disorders and the role of supportive personnel, training in behavior management, and specific instruction in articulatory and language disorders and their remediation. A great portion of the training time was spent in hands-on experience with the programmed materials.

During implementation of the programs, paraprofessionals followed prepared instructions. Materials, equipment, and activities were predetermined, as were the instructional levels and the order in which activities were to be presented. Aides conducted daily individual sessions, and volunteers worked with children twice weekly.

Promising results accrued from the utilization of paraprofessionals. Although children serviced by volunteers did not progress as rapidly as those seen by paid aides, most students improved their linguistic or articulatory skills. The authors concluded that paraprofessionals had been assets to the speech and language programs in the Los Angeles Unified School District.

Alvord (1977) reported on the utilization of aides in the State of Iowa. Children presenting mild to moderate articulatory disorders were serviced by the nine communication aides who, prior to the implementation of the project, had received three days of training. Additional instruction occurred throughout the school year; both training and supervision were done by certified speech-language pathologists.

Not only did the project result in speech gains by the children; it was also found to be cost effective. The researchers discovered that these trained paraprofessionals were as efficient as speech-language pathologists in remediating mild to moderate articulatory defects. In addition, the per-pupil cost of service delivery was cut from $120.00 to $80.00, a reduction of 33.33 percent. Finally, the utilization of communication aides permitted the servicing of more children, as it reduced the case load of the certified speech-language pathologist.

Programmed instruction provided by paraprofessionals was the subject of a project reported on by Costello and Schoen (1978). Participants in the study were 15 children presenting frontal lisps, as well as five paraprofessionals. All of the paraprofessionals were females who had completed at least two years of college. The S-Pack was utilized for programmed teaching.

The fifteen children were assigned to three experimental groups. Group I children received individual instruction from a trained paraprofessional. The auditory and visual stimuli of the S-Pack were presented via videotape. A paraprofessional also administered the program to Group II children; only the auditory portion of the program was presented via tape. In the final condition, a certified speech-language pathologist administered the S-Pack to five children using live voice.

Following administration of the program, it was found that children working with the paraprofessionals progressed as well and as rapidly as those being seen by the certified speech-language pathologist. According to the authors, the paraprofessionals were equally effective in the administration of the S-Pack as the speech-language pathologist. Further, the utilization of audio and videotapes reduced the responsibilities of the aides, while maintaining consistency in program presentation. Innovations of this type permit the speech-language pathologist to service larger populations with greater effectiveness.

Abraham (1977) experimented with the utilization of both parents and paraprofessionals in the habilitation of preschool children with articulatory errors. Specifically, the researcher sought to determine if parents could execute a home program, monitored by a paraprofessional under the supervision of a speech-language pathologist.

Five subjects were involved in the study; all had unintelligible speech. Following evaluation by the speech-language pathologist, paraprofessionals devised home intervention programs for each child. These programs were developed under the supervision of the speech-language pathologist. The purpose of the program was to teach the child correct production of the target phoneme and to facilitate the integration of that phoneme into contextual speech.

Both the paraprofessional and the speech-language pathologist made the first home visit to explain and demonstrate the program to the parent or parents. At that time, the parents executed the procedures, and any deviations were corrected by the speech-language pathologist. Parents were also taught to discriminate between accurate and inaccurate phonemic productions and to record responses. The paraprofessionals assumed responsibility for home visits after the initial contact; the speech-language pathologist assumed the role of consultant. Both home visits and telephone calls were employed by the paraprofessional to maintain contact with the parents.

All five subjects learned to utilize the target phoneme in contextual speech; the time needed for such remediation ranged from 28 days to 225 days, the average being 90 days. Although the parents were instructed to work with the child two to three times daily, it was apparent that this was not always done. Nevertheless, the author suggested that utilization of parents under the supervision of a paraprofessional reduced the involvement of the speech-language pathologist and permitted the latter to provide more direct therapy services.

School Age Children as Supportive Personnel

Two articles dealt with the utilization of older students as paraprofessionals. Evans and Potter (1974) sought to determine if sixth graders could effectively administer the S-Pack to younger children with frontal lisps. Participants in the study were 24 children whose mean age was seven years, seven months. Group I consisted of eight children who received individual programmed instruction (S-Pack) from an experienced speech-language pathologist. The eight Group II students were instructed by a sixth grade pupil who had previously been enrolled in speech therapy. Group III children were seen by a sixth grader with no history of speech defects.

The researchers selected 15 sixth grade tutors to work with the communicatively disordered children. All tutors had normal hearing and speech patterns, were above average in intelligence, and expressed a willingness to participate in the program. Four one-hour group training sessions were held to teach the tutors to administer the S-Pack. Particular emphasis was placed on auditory discrimination. Following completion of training, the tutors conducted 30-minute sessions with the children on three consecutive days. Each tutor was observed for only 10 minutes during the first session; the remainder of the program was administered independently by the tutor.

Statistical analysis of the results of therapy revealed no significant differences among the three groups. All sixth grade students, regardless of whether they had been enrolled in therapy previously, were as effective as the experienced speech-language pathologist. Moreover, the authors reported that the tutors took genuine pride in their accomplishments. Again, participation of paraprofessional tutors permitted the speech-language pathologists additional time to work with children presenting more complex communicative disorders.

Groher (1976) also investigated the participation of older students, with and without articulatory disorders, in the remediation of younger children presenting misarticulations. He further attempted to determine whether involvement in the remedial process would effect change in the articulation of those older students who had speech disorders.

Participants in Groher's study were 48 students, all of whom had normal intelligence and hearing. Of the younger students, who ranged in age from six to eight years and presented articulatory defects, 24 were randomly assigned to three groups of eight. Of the 24 older students, who ranged from 14 to 17 years of age, 16 had articulatory disorders, and the remaining 8 had normal speech. The following group assignments were made:

Group A
- 8 young children with articulatory defects
- 8 older students with normal speech

Group B
- 8 young children with articulatory defects
- 8 older students enrolled in therapy for remediation of articulatory effects

Group C
- 8 young children with articulatory defects
- 8 older children with articulatory defects not scheduled for therapy

The older students met with a speech-language pathologist for a half-hour session once per week; although the session topics varied, they all related to the principles of remediation of articulatory disorders and the application of these principles. Each older student worked with his younger charge for a half hour, twice weekly over a four-month period. Older students in Group B were also seen once weekly for half-hour therapy sessions.

In looking at the pretest and posttest results of the younger children, it was found that Group B students made the greatest gains. Similarly, older Group B students made more improvement than did older Group C subjects. The difference between the two groups was not significant, however. Although the author did not attempt to compare the effectiveness of older students to that of the speech-language pathologist, he was able to determine that, when properly guided, these pupils could effect change in the articulatory patterns of younger children.

In sum, a review of the literature indicates that nonprofessionals have been and are being utilized to assist speech-language pathologists. Those researchers who have reported on projects employing supportive personnel have been guardedly optimistic in their assessment of these programs. Several issues regarding the utilization of paraprofessionals, however, have yet to be determined.

ISSUES SURROUNDING THE UTILIZATION
OF SUPPORTIVE PERSONNEL

As noted in the first section of this chapter, the supportive personnel issue is not a new one. In March 1967, a seminar to discuss the use of such persons was held in Houston, Texas (American Speech and Hearing Association, 1967). Participants included speech-language pathologists as well as professionals from related disciplines who had been involved in developing subprofessional training programs; represented were the fields of nursing, education, psychology, occupational therapy, and dentistry. Each of these representatives discussed their experiences in training and deploying supportive personnel.

Four major topics were considered during the three-day seminar. These included the role that might be played by supportive personnel, the training that should be required, the relationship between the paraprofessional and the supervising speech-language pathologist, and the impact that the utilization of supportive personnel might have on the manpower shortage occurring at that time. Two seminar participants were charged with issuing a complete report of the seminar to the Executive Committee of ASHA. A later report, including recommendations, was also promised.

In the September 1967 issue of *Asha,* the views of a conference participant appeared in a Special Report (Irwin, 1967). The initial concern of the author of the report was the personnel shortage in the area of speech-language pathology and the means of alleviating that problem. Among the solutions cited was the utilization of supportive personnel. Following consideration of paraprofessionals in other disciplines, examples of their utilization in speech pathology and audiology were presented. The author also speculated about problems that might occur when supportive personnel are utilized and raised the following questions:

- Does the term *supportive personnel* refer to paid aides or to volunteers?
- Should the age of the candidate be a consideration?
- Should paraprofessionals have some limited background in speech and hearing? Should they have degrees in other fields?
- Should aides be specifically trained to assist speech-language pathologists or audiologists, or should they be generalists?

- Should supportive personnel be trained to work in all areas of communicative disorders, or should specialization be required?
- Should the position be terminal, or might it be suitable for a preprofessional student in speech-language pathology or audiology?
- Should there be different levels of supportive personnel, so that there is room for advancement?
- Should the standards for paraprofessionals be uniform and, if so, who should establish the standards?

The author also explored such issues as the appropriate title for supportive personnel, their possible organizational affiliations, and their role. An important closing comment related to the effects of supportive personnel on certified speech-language pathologists and on the professional environments in which they function. In this regard, the author discussed the desirable ratio of paraprofessionals to certified professionals, the nature of supervisory practices, and the ethical and legal issues that may arise. In conclusion, the author cautioned that rigid standards, established in haste, might put the profession in an untenable position at some point in the future and that further study would be preferable.

In still another offering, Ptacek (1967) encouraged speech-language pathologists and audiologists to accept the concept of supportive personnel as "an extension of the professional worker's nervous system" (p. 403). He pointed out that paraprofessionals could function in a variety of roles, from housekeeper to reporter to psychotherapist. According to Ptacek, questions to be resolved included the specific functions of supportive personnel, their training, and their qualifications. In addition, he believes it is necessary to determine what training professionals themselves would need in order to use paraprofessionals efficiently. Finally, Ptacek reminded the reader that university professors have been using supportive personnel (graduate and research assistants) for years with good results. With careful selection and training, and with appropriate placement, supportive personnel can function effectively.

In 1969, recommendations from the Committee on Supportive Personnel appointed in 1967 were accepted by the Legislative Council of the American Speech and Hearing Association (American Speech and Hearing Association Committee on Supportive Personnel, 1970). The guidelines recommended by the Committee dealt with the role, training, and supervision of the task-oriented paraprofessional, or "communication aide," who is trained on the job (see Table 9-1).

Norton (1975) was enthusiastic in his support of paraprofessionals. He reported that as of July 1974, a total of 11 states had provisions for licensing supportive personnel. He also said that in the absence of guidelines from ASHA (but note that ASHA guidelines were published in 1970), ruling on the

Table 9-1
Guidelines for the Role, Training,
and Supervision of Communication Aides

Role
- The certified speech-language pathologist musst direct all work done by the communication aide and must assume responsibility for such work.
- The communication aide is prohibited from decision making regarding assessment, intervention, or disposition of clients.
- The communication aides may be assigned only tasks for which they have been trained.
- It is the speech-language pathologist's or audiologist's responsibility to define the aide's roles and duties.
- Equal employment opportunities should be enforced. It is important that candidates be able to communicate effectively, demonstrate empathy for communicatively handicapped individuals, and be able to understand the cultural and linguistic community in which they themselves function.

On-the-job-training
- The training of the communication aide should be task-oriented.
- The selection and training of communication aides should be left to the discretion of the professional worker and/or employing agency.
- The nature and duration of training should be appropriate to the assigned tasks; the employing agency is responsible for providing such training.
- Certified speech-language pathologists or audiologists must provide training for all client-related services.
- Continuing in-service training should be provided to the communication aide by the employing agency.
- Task-oriented training should be provided. The nature of the training must be consistent with the task of the employment setting.
- If necessary, guidance should be provided to the communication aide in the areas of personal work habits, professionalism, and communication.

Supervision
- Communication aides must function only under the direction of a certified speech-language pathologist or audiologist.
- The certified professional has moral, ethical, and legal responsibility for all clients serviced by the communication aide.
- The speech-language pathologist must ensure professional evaluation of each client, must devise an intervention strategy, must maintain contact with the client, and must review the case prior to its termination.
- It is recommended that service agencies utilizing communication aides be registered by the Professional Services Board of the American Board of Examiners in Speech Pathology and Audiology of ASHA.
- The communication aide must not be encouraged to make clinical decisions.
- The ratio of certified personnel to communication aides should not exceed 1:4.

SOURCE: American Speech and Hearing Association Committee on Supportive Personnel, 1970.

qualifications of supportive personnel could be left to agencies other than ASHA. Perhaps because of the perceived inactivity of ASHA, the National Association for Hearing and Speech Action (NAHSA), with funding from the federal government, established pilot programs to train supportive personnel. The program for speech pathologists was initiated in 1973. Candidates were required to be high school graduates, have appropriate communicative abilities, be able to function under supervision, and desire to help communicatively disordered individuals. Instructed by ASHA-certified persons (or individuals with comparable credentials), the applicants were required to complete at least 160 hours of classroom instruction and 244 hours of observation and therapy. Among the subjects covered in classroom instruction were anatomy, neurology, speech and language development, phonetics, and audiology. Applicants were also required to have an understanding of the various communicative disorders.

Once on the job, the speech pathology assistants had such responsibilities and compilation of case histories, execution of therapy for all disorders, maintenance of contact with clients and their families, participation in screenings, and other assigned duties. Independent judgments were not made by the assistants; instead, they carried out the instructions of the speech-language pathologists.

Norton cited several advantages in the use of paraprofessionals. According to him, the availability of an assistant permits the speech pathologist time to attend conferences or parent meetings. Additionally, services to the communicatively handicapped can be expanded. Finally, he anticipated that the utilization of speech pathology assistants would increase once the benefits of their services were realized.

Moll (1974) pursued the issue of supportive personnel in an *Asha* "Special Report." Noting that the original thrust for paraprofessionals came from a manpower shortage, he suggested that a misdistribution of qualified speech-language pathologists might continue even after the supply met the demand. An additional motivating factor was the need for economical service delivery. Second, Moll acknowledged that supportive personnel were being used increasingly, working under various titles in diverse employment settings. With pressure for supportive personnel continuing to be exerted by governmental agencies and with state regulations in place for the recognition of such individuals, Moll suggested that additional policies and guidelines be established.

The ASHA guidelines, according to Moll, offer extreme flexibility in role definition, training, and utilization. Although flexibility is desirable in some cases, a number of disadvantages are apparent. Horizontal mobility for the paraprofessional, for example, is not ensured. Further, the establishment of recognized occupational classifications is not possible under the ASHA guidelines. The training of supportive personnel is also a consideration.

ASHA specifies that its guidelines pertain to task-oriented, on-the-job training. Moll suggests that formal classroom training might be required if more specific job categories were established. Finally, the question of vertical mobility is addressed. Should opportunities for advancement as paraprofessionals be provided, or should the position be considered a "dead-end" proposition? These questions have far-reaching implications. Moll, in concluding his report, expressed the opinion that specific categories of supportive personnel should be established, and that opportunities for both horizontal and vertical mobility should be provided.

DISCUSSION

The foregoing discussions reflect some of the issues surrounding the utilization of supportive personnel. A review of the literature suggests almost complete agreement regarding the effectiveness of such persons, whether they be mothers, students in training, high school graduates, or retrained aides. Unfortunately for the objective reader, reports of the unsuccessful utilization of paraprofessionals may not have appeared in the professional journals.

With regard to whether supportive personnel should be utilized, the answer seems to be a qualified affirmative. The reservations are related to the task, training, and personal qualifications of the individual paraprofessional, as well as the attitudes and preparation of the supervising speech-language pathologist. Regarding the tasks assigned to supportive personnel, the general trend is to assign specific steps of articulation therapy to the paraprofessional; teaching the target phoneme is usually not included. Several researchers report the successful utilization of supportive personnel in language therapy and in drill work with the hearing impaired. Individuals implementing such therapy have received either task-oriented training or task-oriented training supplemented by formal course work. The training, entry qualifications, and titles of these persons have varied. One way of resolving these differences, as Moll has indicated, may be to follow the lead taken by other professions and create tiers of supportive personnel. For the purposes of this discussion, only two levels are considered: the task-oriented tier (Level I) and the task-oriented tier that includes formal classroom preparation (Level II).

The personal entry qualifications for Level I and Level II would be similar. Candidates should have hearing within normal limits and adequate written and oral communication skills. They should be sensitive to the needs of communicatively disordered individuals and capable of dealing with persons presenting such problems in an objective manner. Further, applicants should be able to relate to the supervising speech-language pathologist and other professional workers and be willing to accept constructive criticism. The final selection of candidates should be made by the supervising speech-language pathologist based on the perceived needs of the clients and the abilities of the paraprofessional.

Most agencies or individuals establishing educational qualifications for paraprofessionals have cited a high school diploma as requisite. There is considerable evidence that possessing a high school diploma does not necessarily indicate any specific level of achievement and, therefore, may not serve as a discriminating qualification. Evidence of appropriate oral, written, and mathematic skills might be a better educational criterion. Additional competency requirements would vary depending on the specific job description. Level II personnel, for example, who were to work with language disordered, mentally retarded children would profit from course work in language development, language disorders, and characteristics of the retarded population. Competence in the use of specific language programs might also be required. The development of appropriate curricula would be the joint responsibility of the various agencies and a university department of speech-language pathology and audiology; a team instructional approach might be employed. If such specializations were available at Level II, educational background consistent with these specializations would be desirable.

The training of Level I and Level II personnel would differ, also. Both tiers of personnel would be given an orientation to the specific job setting and instruction in the responsibilities peculiar to that environment. Level I persons would receive appropriate task-oriented training, particularly in the area of articulation therapy. Supportive personnel at the second level would also receive instruction in the implementation of therapeutic programs, but a broader spectrum of intervention tools would be included. The training of all supportive personnel should be the responsibility of the supervising speech-language pathologist or employing agency.

With regard to the actual responsibilities of supportive personnel, flexibility is important. Research suggests that clerical duties, maintenance of materials and equipment, and execution of articulation therapy are tasks commonly assigned to paraprofessionals. Level II personnel might also be able to compile case history information, serve as monitors and reporters of communicative behavior outside of the therapy setting, and participate in the implementation of language programs. If specialization within the Level II category were available, limited expansion into other areas of communicative disorders might be possible. Again, the duties of the supportive personnel would be determined by the supervising speech-language pathologist, who would assume all ethical, moral, and legal responsibilities to the clients for any work done by the paraprofessional.

A final consideration concerns the qualifications of the supervising speech-language pathologist. Minimally, that person should have a master's degree and several years of experience. Included in his or her training should be some background in supervisory techniques. The supervising speech-language pathologist should also have an understanding of the role of the paraprofessional, respect that role, and be supportive of the concept. Speech-language pathologists who feel threatened by supportive personnel will probably be inefficient in the utilization of such persons. Finally, the supervising speech-language pathologist must be capable of assigning tasks commensurate with the abilities of paraprofessionals and monitoring their work objectively.

The advantages of using supportive personnel have been discussed throughout this section. The most frequently cited advantage is that the certified speech-language pathologist is able to concentrate on providing quality services to children with complex problems, while the supportive person assumes responsibility of routine articulation therapy and housekeeping chores. Possible disadvantages include the professional time expended in orientation and supervision of the paraprofessional. There is also an inherent risk that the supportive person might assume more responsibility than he or she is capable of handling; prevention of this eventuality, however, is the responsibility of the supervising speech-language pathologist. Finally, some speech-language pathologists have expressed the fear that school districts might employ supportive personnel rather than professionals. It has been shown that trained subprofessionals can execute articulation programs and even language habilitation as efficiently as certified persons. Little evidence exists, however, that supportive personnel can deal effectively with individuals who stutter, have vocal disorders, or display multiple communicative disorders. Perhaps a redefinition of the role of the professional speech-language pathologist is necessary; in such a definition, the reponsibilities of the paraprofessional should be included, since it appears that they are a part of the present and will be a part of the future.

REFERENCES

Abraham, V. Parents as articulation therapists. *The Illinois Speech and Hearing Association Journal,* 1977, *10,* 19–22.

Alpiner, J. G., Ogden, J. A., & Wiggins, J. E. The utilization of supportive personnel in speech correction in the public schools: A pilot project. *Asha,* 1970, *12,* 599–604.

Alvord, D. J. Innovation in speech therapy: A cost effective program. *Exceptional Children,* 1977, *43,* 520–525.

American Speech and Hearing Association Committee on Supportive Personnel. Guidelines on the role, training, and supervision of the communication aide. *Asha,* 1970, *12,* 78–80.

American Speech and Hearing Association. Seminar on supportive personnel. *Asha,* 1967, *9,* 140–141.

Braunstein, M. S. Communication aide: A pilot project. *Language, Speech, and Hearing Services in Schools,* 1972, *3,* 32–35.

Bush, C., & Bonachea, M. Parental involvement in language development: The PAL program. *Language, Speech, and Hearing Services in Schools,* 1973, *4,* 82–85.

Carpenter, R. L., & Augustine, L. E. A pilot training program for parent–clinicians. *Journal of Speech and Hearing Disorders,* 1973, *38,* 48–57.

Carrier, J. K., Jr. A program of articulation therapy administered by mothers. *Journal of Speech and Hearing Disorders,* 1970, *35,* 344–353.

Costello, J., & Schoen, J. The effectiveness of paraprofessionals and a speech clinician as agents of articulation intervention using programmed instruction. *Language, Speech, and Hearing Services in Schools,* 1978, *9,* 118–128.

Evans, C. M., & Potter, R. E. The effectiveness of the S-Pack when administered by sixth grade children to primary-grade children. *Language, Speech, and Hearing Services in Schools,* 1974, *5,* 85–90.

Fudula, J. B., England, G., & Ganoung L. Utilization of Parents in a Speech Correction Program. *Exceptional Children,* 1972, *38,* 407–412.

Galloway, H. F., Jr., & Blue, C. M. Paraprofessional personnel in articulation therapy. *Language, Speech, and Hearing Services in Schools,* 1975, *6,* 125–130.

Gray, B. B., & Barker, K. Use of aides in an articulation therapy program. *Exceptional Children,* 1977, *43,* 534–536.

Groher, M. The experimental use of cross-age relationships in public school speech remediation. *Language, Speech, and Hearing Services in Schools,* 1976, *7,* 250–258.

Guess, D., Smith J. O., & Ensminger, E. E. The role of nonprofessional persons in teaching language skills to mentally retarded children. *Exceptional Children,* 1971, *37,* 447–453.

Hall, P. K., & Knutson, C. L. The use of preprofessional students as communication aides in the schools. *Language, Speech, and Hearing Services in Schools,* 1978, *9,* 162–168.

Irwin, J. V. Supportive personnel in speech pathology and audiology. *Asha,* 1967, *9,* 348–354.

Lillywhite, H. Make mother a clinician. *Journal of Speech and Hearing Disorders,* 1948, *13,* 61–66.

MacDonald, J. D., Blott, J. P., Gordon, K., Spiegel, B., & Hartmann, M. An experimental parent-assisted treatment program for preschool language-delayed children. *Journal of Speech and Hearing Disorders,* 1974, *39,* 395–415.

Moll, K. L. Issues facing us—Supportive personnel. *Asha,* 1974, *16,* 357–358.

Norton, D. E. Try them—You'll like them. *Hearing and Speech Action,* 1975, *43,* 10–11.

Ptacek, P. Supportive personnel as an extension of the professional worker's nervous system. *Asha,* 1967, *9,* 403–405.

Scalero, A. M., & Eskenazi, C. The use of supportive personnel in a public school speech and language program. *Language, Speech, and Hearing Services in Schools,* 1976, *7,* 150–158.

Sommers, R. K. Factors in effectiveness of mothers trained to aid in speech correction. *Journal of Speech and Hearing Disorders,* 1962, *27,* 178–186.

Sommers, R. K., Schilling, S. P., Paul, C. D., Copetas, F. G., Bowser, D. C., & McClintock, C. J. Training parents of children with functional misarticulations. *Journal of Speech and Hearing Research,* 1959, *2,* 258–265.

Sommers, R. K., Furlong, A. K., Rhodes, F. E., Fichter, G. R., Bowser, D. C., Copetas, F. G., & Saunders, Z. G. Effects of maternal attitude upon improvement in articulation when mothers are trained to assist in speech correction. *Journal of Speech and Hearing Disorders,* 1964, *29,* 126–132.

Strong, B. Public school speech technicians in Minnesota. *Language, Speech, and Hearing Services in Schools,* 1972, *3,* 53–56.

Tufts, L. C., & Holliday, A. R. Effectiveness of trained parents as speech therapists. *Journal of Speech and Hearing Disorders,* 1959, *24,* 395–401.

Wing, D. M., & Heimgartener, L. M. Articulation carry-over procedure implemented by parents. *Language, Speech, and Hearing Services in Schools,* 1973, *4,* 182–195.

Wingo, J. W. Student spech and hearing "teams" in the public school. *Asha,* 1970, *12,* 605–606.

10

Epilogue

"Men have forgotten this truth," said the fox, "but you must not forget it. You become responsible, forever, for what you have tamed. *

Throughout this text I have tried to avoid expressing personal opinions and biases, and I hope my effort has been successful. This book is not intended to be a "how-to" manual, but a "what's-possible" text. It is difficult, however, to discuss the subject of public school speech-language pathology services without creating some reactions. Those of you reading this text should have positive feelings about a career in public schools. There was a time when working in such an environment was somewhat tedious; physical needs were not always met, equipment was inadequate, and materials were in short supply. Moreover, the children seen by the speech-language pathologist either presented "garden variety" articulatory defects or exhibited problems (specifically in the area of language) that the professional was unprepared to handle. Today, some of these same problems may still exist, but contemporary school speech-language pathologists are better equipped, have more sensitive testing tools and materials, and have training and experience that have prepared them to work effectively with children presenting a variety of problems. With the advent of state and federal legislation that requires that all handicapped children must have access to a free, appropriate education in the least restrictive environment, there is little doubt that the public school setting

---

*From *The Little Prince* by Antoine De Saint-Exupéry. New York: Harcourt, Brace and Company, 1943, p. 71. Reprinted by permission of Harcourt Brace Jovanovich, Inc.

presents a tremendous challenge to speech-language pathologists. In this brief final chapter, as a means of summarizing the text, I will permit myself the luxury of offering some personal observations about public school speech-language services.

The first chapter of the book dealt with historical aspects of the profession, qualifications of public school personnel, and professional titles. Little comment is needed on the origins of the profession, but the last two topics should be thought provoking. A question still to be answered is whether the preparation of school personnel should differ from the preservice preparation of students who plan to work in other settings. As of this date, the American Speech-Language-Hearing Association (ASHA) has not generated a certificate for public school personnel, although other areas of specific certification are under consideration. States are in some disagreement about requirements for certification; perhaps speech-language pathologists in the midwest require more education courses to function effectively in the schools than their counterparts in the south. Uniformity in certification requirements throughout the states would certainly facilitate the mobility of school speech-language pathologists and decrease the problems of preservice academic advisement. With regard to the professional title used by speech-language pathologists in the schools, the ASHA-designated title has been employed throughout this text. As stated in Chapter 1, this does not indicate approval of the title. Not only is it cumbersome for use in the school setting, it is also somewhat difficult to include a — (dash) in oral conversation. Thus, speech-language pathologist becomes "speech (pause) language pathologist" or "speechlanguagepathologist." It is interesting that a profession that deals with oral communication has a title that is not easily communicated orally. If given a choice of titles, it would seem that "speech and language clinician" might be preferable to "speech-language pathologist." All areas of disorders would be included and less imposing terminology would be employed. Unfortunately, what professionals choose to call themselves is sometimes irrelevant in the school setting; school "speech-language pathologists" may still be "speech teachers" or, when spoken by children with articulatory disorders, "peech teacher."

Chapter 2 considered state and federal legislation involving the education of handicapped children. There is little doubt that such legislation has contributed to public awareness of the problems of the handicapped and has improved the quality and quantity of services provided to them. These laws have also produced anxiety among professionals, and wrinkles must still be ironed out. PL 94-142 requirements present some procedural difficulties needing resolution. It is possible that modifications within the law will be made even before this book goes into print. These changes, it is hoped, will serve to strengthen the regulations while reducing unnecessary burdens on professionals. The reader is cautioned to remain abreast of such modifications, now and in the future, in order to function knowledgeably within the school system.

Although it was noted that personal biases were unintentional, it is likely that the reader detected some expression of opinion in Chapter 3. Screening seems to be the preferred method of case finding at the elementary schools level; teacher referral is more popular in secondary schools. When employing screening techniques, it is important that the speech-language pathologist be realistic in identifying children with communicative disorders. Some students with minor problems may not be handicapped in the layperson's judgment; they are handicapped only in the eyes (and/or ears) of the speech-language pathologist. Many famous individuals (including politicians and newscasters) have been successful in spite of nonstandard communicative styles. Once children have been carefully identified as having suspected communicative disorders, evaluative procedures must be chosen sensibly. Numerous tools are available for the formal testing of such children, but the wise speech-language pathologist will make extensive use of clinical judgment. Observation of the child and analysis of language and speech samples must comprise the better portion of the diagnostic. As many of you know, not all individuals respond well to formal testing, and it is the application of communicative abilities in "real life" situations that should be considered.

Chapter 4 considered case selection and management alternatives. Certainly the reader became aware that not all professionals are in agreement regarding case selection priorities; however, it is hoped that sufficient information was provided to encourage the development of personal philosophies. Regarding management alternatives, it is possible and even probable that many speech-language pathologists in the schools do not have access to some of the options presented. When this is the case, it is necessary to select the most appropriate therapy delivery system available and then to provide evidence to administrators that other options are required.

Scheduling models were discussed in Chapter 5. Although evidence was presented to support the effectiveness of various block systems in the modification of articulatory errors, intermittent systems continue to enjoy greater popularity. The needs of the individual child are to be considered in scheduling; ideally, children with articulatory disorders should be seen for intensive cycle therapy for blocks of time, and children with other types of communicative problems should receive intensive therapy throughout the school year. The reader will soon learn, however, that ideal scheduling is not always possible in schools or other settings. Therefore, inadequate as it may seem in many cases, intermittent therapy is preferable to intensive cycle scheduling when a choice must be made. A combination of both is an attractive compromise.

IEPs need little comment. Even though IEP requirements are presenting difficulties to school speech-language pathologists, they have been accepted as a necessary part of PL 94-142 compliance. It is hoped that the specimen IEP forms presented in Chapter 6 will assist the reader in the preparation of such programs.

Chapter 7 considered service delivery. Many areas of intervention could have been discussed in this section, but the constraints of space, the intent of the text, and the concerns of the author restricted the discussion to service delivery to culturally different children, youths confined to correctional institutions, and high school students. Students in training are exposed to children and adults presenting disorders of articulation, voice, fluency, language, and hearing, but they may be less aware of the problems presented by culturally different populations. Philosophical decisions based on sound evidence should assist the student in dealing with such individuals. As was indicated in this chapter, there is limited evidence for the need for speech-language services in secondary schools or in institutions for juvenile delinquents. Students must prepare, however, to work with adolescents, and it is hoped that the brief introduction included in this chapter will motivate preservice speech-language pathologists to seek additional information.

The speech-language pathologist wears many hats during the execution of his or her responsibilities. Administration, service delivery, and participation in the team approach were discussed throughout the text. That the public school speech-language pathologist may participate in research seems almost a redundancy; each day in the life of a school speech-language pathologist is full of opportunities for research. Contributions to *Language, Speech, and Hearing Services in Schools* bear witness to the fact that many school professionals are now allocating time to prepare and share the results of their research. Responsibilities that are now gaining prominence are those involved in counseling and supervision, topics on which Chapter 8 focused attention. Many school speech-language pathologists have had little formal exposure to counseling techniques; many learned to counsel parents and clients simply by counseling parents and clients. But the results were sometimes disastrous. Similarly, supervision was a responsibility professionals first assumed when student teachers were assigned to them. On-the-job training was necessary. Today's speech-language pathologists should be aware that these are responsibilities that they must assume, and it behooves students in training to seek adequate preparation for these roles.

Chapter 9 dealt with a somewhat sensitive issue facing the profession—the utilization of supportive personnel. Parents are considered important in habilitative-rehabilitative efforts, but they are viewed as nonthreatening. Paid supportive personnel, on the other hand, pose serious threats to certified professionals in the schools. The successful utilization of paraprofessionals is documented in the literature. The question that concerns school speech-language pathologists is whether supportive personnel might be employed to the exclusion of certified professionals. Again, the literature suggests that paraprofessionals, carefully trained and supervised, can be successful in working with children with articulatory defects and linguistic problems. There is little evidence, however, to support the utilization of paraprofessionals with other groups of communicatively disordered children. When the speech-language pathologist is instrumental in selecting, training, and supervising supportive personnel, it appears that the latter can be important factors in efficient service delivery.

This book began as a rather modest project. It has evolved into a text that will, I hope, help prepare school speech-language pathologists to function effectively within the system.

Index

a
b
c
d
e
f
g
h
1 i
8 2 j